MINIMALLY INVASIVE GYNECOLOGY SERIES

Management of Ectopic Pregnancy

Management of Ectopic Pregnancy

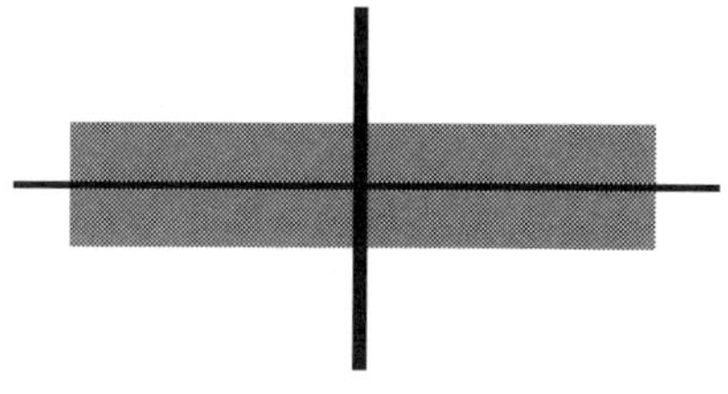

edited by

Richard E. Leach, MD
Associate Professor
Department of Obstetrics and Gynecology
Division of Reproductive Endocrinology and Infertility
Wayne State University School of Medicine
Detroit, Michigan

Steven J. Ory, MD
Clinical Associate Professor
Department of Obstetrics and Gynecology
University of Miami;
Northwest Center for Infertility and Reproductive Endocrinology
Margate, Florida

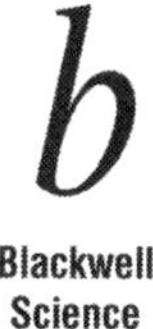

Blackwell Science

Editorial Offices:
Commerce Place, 350 Main Street, Malden, Massachusetts 02148, USA
Osney Mead, Oxford OX2 0EL, England
25 John Street, London WC1N 2BL, England
23 Ainslie Place, Edinburgh EH3 6AJ, Scotland
54 University Street, Carlton, Victoria 3053, Australia

Other Editorial Offices:
Blackwell Wissenschafts-Verlag GmbH, Kurfürstendamm 57, 10707 Berlin, Germany
Blackwell Science KK, MG Kodenmacho Building, 7-10 Kodenmacho Nihombashi, Chuo-ku, Tokyo 104, Japan

Distributors:
USA
   Blackwell Science, Inc.
   Commerce Place
   350 Main Street
   Malden, Massachusetts 02148
   (Telephone orders: 800-215-1000 or 781-388-8250; fax orders: 781-388-8270)
Canada
   Login Brothers Book Company
   324 Saulteaux Crescent
   Winnipeg, Manitoba, R3J 3T2
   (Telephone orders: 204-224-4068)
Australia
   Blackwell Science Pty, Ltd.
   54 University Street
   Carlton, Victoria 3053
   (Telephone orders: 03-9347-0300;
   fax orders: 03-9349-3016)
Outside North America and Australia
   Blackwell Science, Ltd.
   c/o Marston Book Services, Ltd.
   P.O. Box 269
   Abingdon
   Oxon OX14 4YN
   England
   (Telephone orders: 44-01235-465500;
   fax orders: 44-01235-465555)

Notice: The indications and dosages of all drugs in this book have been recommended in the medical literature and conform to the practices of the general medical community. The indications described do not necessarily have specific approval by the U. S. Food and Drug Administration for use in the diseases and dosages for which they are recommended. The package insert for each drug should be consulted for use and dosage as approved by the FDA. Because standards for usage change, it is advisable to keep abreast of revised recommendations, particularly those concerning new drugs.

Acquisitions: Christopher Davis
Development: Karin Commeret
Production: Kevin Sullivan
Manufacturing: Lisa Flanagan
Cover design by Leslie Haimes
Typeset by Laser Words
Printed and bound by Braun-Brumfield, Inc.

Printed in the United States of America
00 01 02 03 5 4 3 2 1

The Blackwell Science logo is a trade mark of Blackwell Science Ltd., registered at the United Kingdom Trade Marks Registry

Library of Congress Cataloging-in-Publication Data

Management of ectopic pregnancy / edited by Richard E. Leach, Steven
   J. Ory.
      p.   cm.
   ISBN 0-632-04469-1
   1. Ectopic Pregnancy — Treatment.   2. Pregnancy — Complications.
 I. Leach, Richard E.   II. Ory, Steven J.
   [DNLM: 1. Pregnancy, Ectopic — therapy.   WQ 220 M266   2000]
 RG586.M36   2000
 618.3'1 — dc21
 DNLM/DLC
 for Library of Congress   99-16453
                                                   CIP

Contents

Contributors

Ricardo Azziz, MD, MPH
Professor of Obstetrics and
  Gynecology, and Medicine
Division of Reproductive Biology
The University of Alabama at
  Birmingham
Birmingham, Alabama

John R. Brumsted, MD
Professor and Director of
  Reproductive Endocrinology and
  Infertility
Head, Section of Gynecology
University of Vermont College of
  Medicine
Burlington, Vermont

Michael P. Diamond, MD
Director, Division of Reproductive
  Endocrinology and Infertility
Kamran S. Moghissi Professor,
  Department of Obstetrics and
  Gynecology
Wayne State University School of
  Medicine;
Detroit Medical Center
Detroit, Michigan

Edward C. Ditkoff, MD
Assistant Professor
Department of Obstetrics and
  Gynecology
Columbia University
College of Physicians and Surgeons
New York, New York

Samuel C. Johnson, MD
Assistant Professor of Radiology
Wayne State University Medical
  School;
Vice-Chief, Department of Radiology
Hutzel Hospital
Detroit, Michigan

Richard E. Leach, MD
Associate Professor, Department of
  Obstetrics and Gynecology
Division of Reproductive
  Endocrinology and Infertility
Wayne State University School of
  Medicine
Detroit, Michigan

Steven J. Ory, MD
Clinical Associate Professor
Department of Obstetrics and
  Gynecology
University of Miami
Miami, Florida;
Northwest Center for Infertility and
  Reproductive Endocrinology
Margate, Florida

Nilsa C. Ramirez, MD
Department of Pathology and
  Laboratory Medicine
Spectrum Health
Grand Rapids, Michigan

Mark V. Sauer, MD
Professor and Chief
Division of Reproductive
  Endocrinology
Department of Obstetrics and
  Gynecology
Columbia University
College of Physicians and
  Surgeons
New York, New York

Scott Slayden, MD
Assistant Professor
Department of Obstetrics and
  Gynecology
Medical College of Georgia
Augusta, Georgia

Thomas G. Stovall, MD
Professor and Vice Chairman
Department of Obstetrics and
  Gynecology
Clinical Chief of Women's Health
  Services
University of Tennessee, Memphis,
  College of Medicine
Memphis, Tennessee

Togas Tulandi, MD
Professor of Obstetrics and
  Gynecology
Director, Division of Reproductive
  Endocrinology and Infertility
McGill University
Montreal, Quebec
Canada

Preface

Physicians who care for women during their reproductive years are challenged to identify those women at risk for ectopic pregnancy and to subsequently diagnose them in a timely fashion. The failure to do so may result in serious mortality and morbidity. According to one study, in over half of the maternal deaths due to ectopic pregnancy, a physician saw the patient during the preceding 48 hours (1). The purpose of this book is to provide a concise office reference on the diagnosis and treatment of ectopic pregnancies.

The availability of sensitive serum human chorionic gonadotropin (hCG) assays, transvaginal ultrasonography, and liberal use of laparoscopy have led to the earlier diagnosis of ectopic pregnancy, often before hemorrhage and tubal rupture. As a result of these advances, we are encountering ectopic pregnancies along a continuum of their natural course. For example, early ectopic pregnancies have subtle differences from later ectopic pregnancies both in their ability to be detected and in options for treatment, which range from expectant management to salpingectomy.

This collection of chapters from some of the leading experts on the topic of ectopic pregnancy provides a resource to the physician often faced with these diagnostic and therapeutic questions. *Management of Ectopic Pregnancy* addresses the incidence of ectopic pregnancy and the impact of ambulatory treatment on the accuracy of the data. Risk factors are discussed, providing useful information to the clinician to triage patients at risk by appropriate active surveillance for pregnancy location. The chapter on histopathology contrasts eutopic and ectopic chorionic villi histology and their relation to the decidua and tubal mucosa, respectively. Discussions of hCG, other serum markers, and transvaginal ultrasound include novel information to support various diagnostic strategies. The information presented on the medical and surgical treatment of ectopic pregnancy is a useful guide to the various treatment modalities that are currently available and their indications. The chapter on the reproductive outcome of treated ectopic pregnancies includes important information to know when counseling patients on future reproductive performance, often a primary concern. Cost analysis and the economic impact of ectopic pregnancy on the health care industry are discussed, with the conclusion that prevention and early diagnosis would result in the largest savings.

It was a privilege for us to serve as co-editors of *Management of Ectopic Pregnancy* and to work with the leading investigators in this area. We trust this book will provide the physician with the understanding of which patients are at risk for ectopic pregnancy and the diagnostic and treatment modalities available for early intervention.

REL

SJO

REFERENCES

1. Ansbacher R, Mills E, Thrush H, Stevenson L. Ectopic pregnancy and maternal mortality in Michigan. Am J Gyn Hem 1989;3:118–126.

1

Ectopic Pregnancy:
Trends and Risks

Richard E. Leach

The number of ectopic pregnancies (EPs) has dramatically increased since the first data on EPs were reported in 1970 (1). The number of hospitalizations for EP, for example, increased from 17,800 in 1970 to 88,400 in 1989 (Fig. 1.1). During this time period, nearly 1 million EP events occurred; the rate of EP per 1000 reported pregnancies showed a fourfold increase, jumping from 4.5 in 1970 to 16 in 1989 (2). On a more hopeful note, the case-fatality rate declined from 35.5 deaths per 10,000 EPs in 1970 to 3.8 deaths per 10,000 EPs in 1989 (Fig. 1.2). Despite this favorable outcome, however, EP represented only 1.6% of all pregnancies in 1989 but was associated with 13% of all pregnancy-related deaths during the first trimester; it is therefore the leading cause of maternal mortality.

An understanding of these trends requires a more detailed elucidation of the methods used for data collection and reporting of results. Characterizing these trends and understanding the risk factors involved will allow the physician to identify those women at risk for EP and to plan earlier intervention, which presumably will decrease morbidity and mortality related to this condition.

The enormous effort by investigators at the Centers for Disease Control and Prevention (CDC) is clearly responsible for our improved understanding of the epidemiology of EP. The CDC's National Hospital

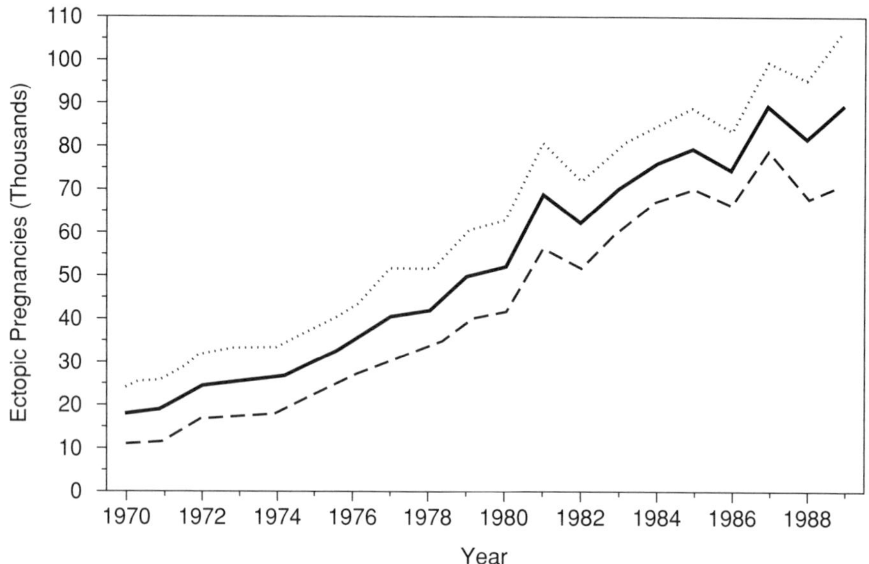

FIG. 1.1.

Estimation of the number of ectopic pregnancies, United States, 1970–1989. Dashed lines represent the upper and lower limits of 95% confidence intervals.

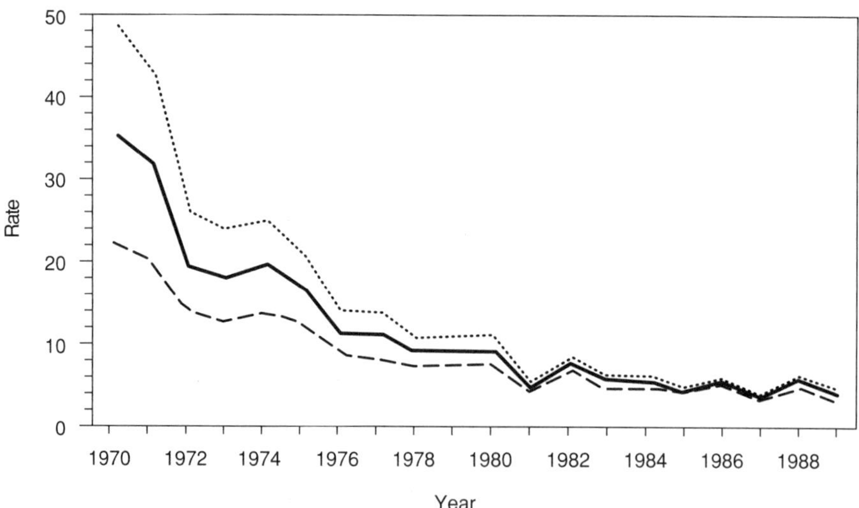

FIG. 1.2.

Rates of ectopic pregnancy mortality, United States, 1970–1989. Data are per 10,000 ectopic pregnancies. Dashed lines represent the upper and lower limits of 95% confidence intervals.

Discharge Survey (NHDS) has assiduously collected data on EP over the past three decades.

Prior to 1988, data from 400 hospitals that responded to NHDS were used to estimate the incidence of EP within geographical regions. Estimates were based on discharge diagnosis and procedure codes abstracted from sample medical records. In 1988, the NHDS surveyed all hospitals with more than 1000 beds or greater than 40,000 annual discharges. ICD-8 code 631 and ICD-9 code 633 were abstracted from medical records for the periods 1970–1978 and 1979–1989, respectively. To calculate EP rates, the number of EPs was divided by the total estimated pregnancies (defined as the sum of live births, legal pregnancy terminations, and EPs). EP-related maternal mortality was estimated from vital statistics collected by NHDS.

In 1990, an additional source of EP data was added to the NHDS-gathered data in an effort to capture those patients with EP not admitted to the hospital. These estimates, which were obtained from the CDC's National Hospital Ambulatory Medical Care Survey (NHAMCS), accounted for those patients treated in the ambulatory surgical setting, but not women treated in a physician's office with medical therapy or asymptomatic patients followed expectantly. This new approach to epidemiology may explain the decline in EP noted since 1988, when conservative therapy was practiced.

During the period 1970–1989, EP rates were higher for African Americans than for Caucasians among all age groups (Fig. 1.3). EP increased with age in both racial groups, with Caucasian and African American women aged 35–44 found to be 3.1 and 3.7 times more likely to experience EP, respectively, than those aged 15–24. During the 1970–1989 period, the risk of death from EP was 3.4 times higher for African Americans than for Caucasians and nearly 5 times higher for African American teenagers than for their Caucasian counterparts (Figs. 1.4 and 1.5). In the United States, the highest rates of total EP occurred in the South, with the highest rates for African Americans and Caucasians occurring in the Midwest and West, respectively.

The number of EP-related hospitalizations decreased to 64,000 in 1990, 54,100 in 1991, and 58,200 in 1992, according to NHDS estimates (Fig. 1.6). The total EP incidence, however, reached 108,800 in 1992

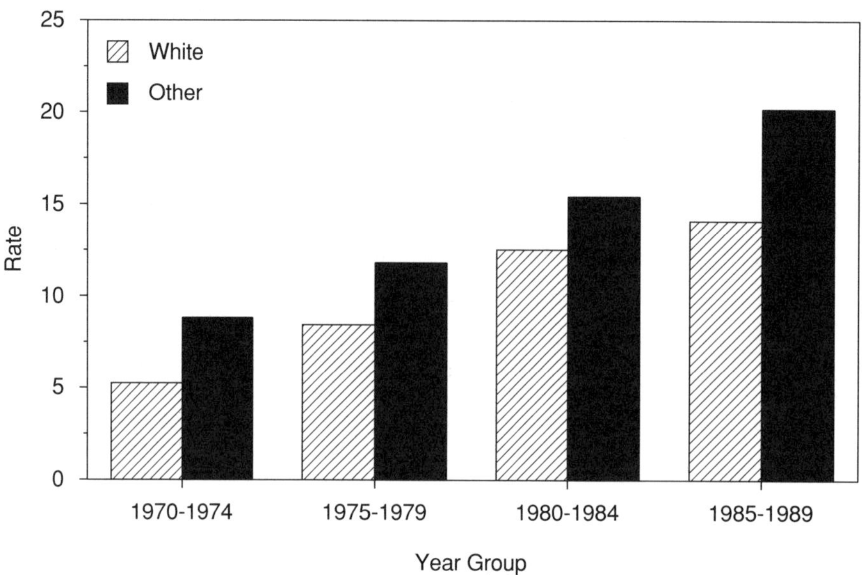

FIG. 1.3.

Rates of ectopic pregnancy by race, United States, 1970–1989. Data are per 1000 reported pregnancies (including live births, legal abortions, and ectopic pregnancies).

according to NHDS and NHAMCS estimates, for a rate of 19.7 EPs per 1000 pregnancies. These more accurate estimates show a continuation of the alarming increases in EP rates seen from 1970 to 1989, even though they still do not account for those patients treated nonsurgically. On the other hand, EP-related mortality continues to decline: EP-related deaths accounted for 9% of maternal deaths in 1992, down from 15% and 13% in 1988 and 1989, respectively.

The rise in EP incidence has placed a greater impetus on understanding behaviors that place a woman at risk for EP. This knowledge may provide an additional means of identifying patients who might benefit from early monitoring for pregnancy location and expediting interventions that would prevent death, decrease morbidity, and minimize health care costs. Although the etiology of EP remains unclear, it appears to stem from both maternal and embryonic factors.

Many of the maternal factors can, theoretically, be attributed to adverse effects on normal fallopian tube anatomy and function. The

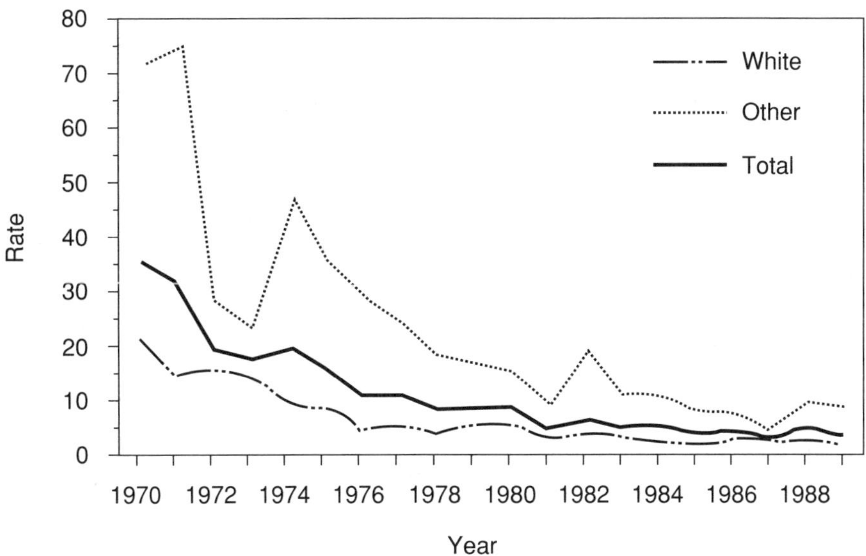

FIG. 1.4.

Rates of ectopic pregnancy mortality by race, United States, 1970–1989. Data are per 10,000 ectopic pregnancies.

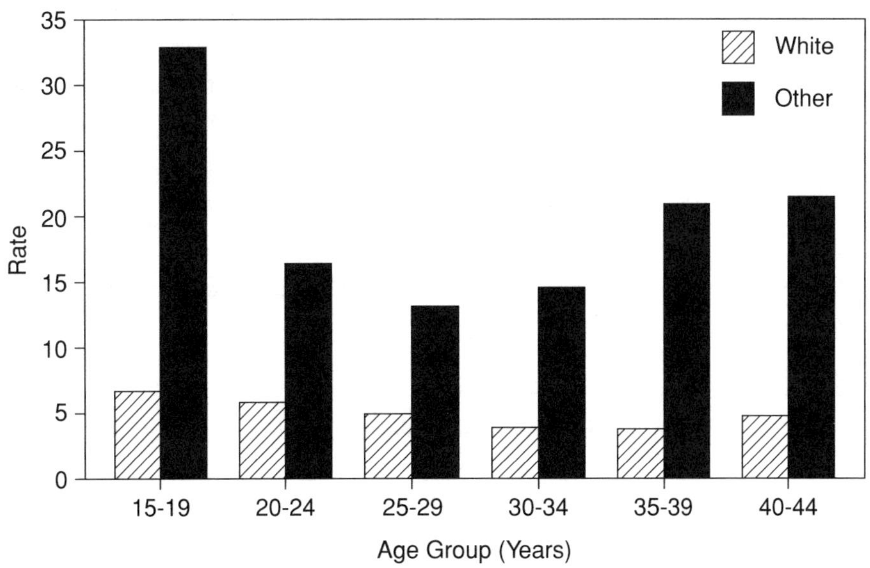

FIG. 1.5.

Case = fatality rates for ectopic pregnancy by race and age group, United States, 1970–1989. Data are per 10,000 ectopic pregnancies.

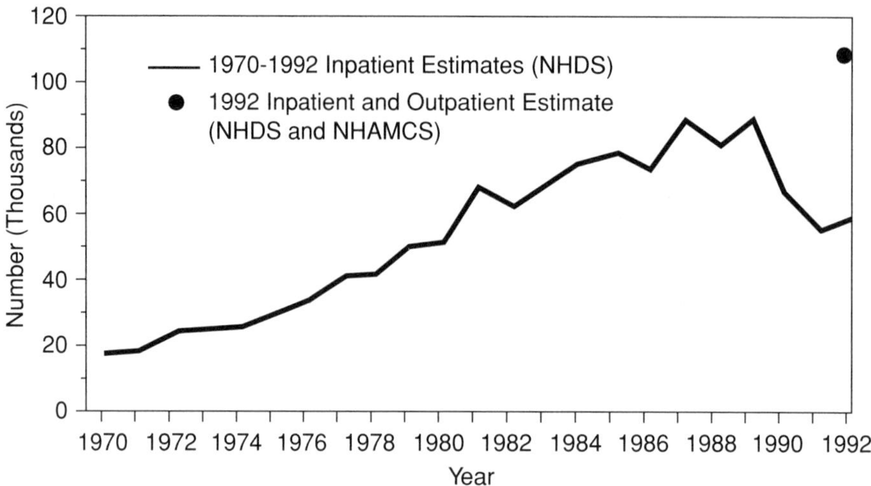

FIG. 1.6.

Number of ectopic pregnancies, United States, 1970–1992. NHDS = National Hospital Discharge Survey; NHAMCS = National Hospital Ambulatory Medical Care Survey.

traditional methods of fallopian tube evaluation rely on gross visual evaluations — either by inspection at surgery or by hysterosalpingography. Newer techniques of tuboscopy promise to provide more accurate tubal mucosal imaging and correlate well with fecundity. Such an approach can better predict tubal function and successful pregnancy. Currently, it remains unclear as to whether compromised tubal function after surgery reflects a preexisting undiagnosed infectious process responsible for the infertility, presumed to be the indication for the surgery, or if it is the direct result of the surgery.

RISK FACTORS

Pelvic Inflammatory Disease

Among women with pelvic inflammatory disease (PID), 5% will experience an ectopic pregnancy, 10% will become infertile, 15% will have chronic pelvic pain, and 25% will develop recurrent infection (3). Studies that diagnosed PID via laparoscopy and graded the infection on a scale of "mild," "moderate," and "severe" (including the presence of a tubo-ovarian abscess) found that 42% of pregnancies following a diagnosis of severe PID are tubal (4,5). Preliminary studies using salpingoscopy, which permits laparoscopic evaluation of the folds of the tubal mucosa, noted that the presence of intraluminal adhesions is associated with an increased risk of ectopic pregnancy (6).

Recurrence

EP is associated with a 12% to 20% recurrence rate (7,8). An 11-year follow-up of 106 women treated for two ectopic pregnancies, 50 of whom desired future fertility, found that 52% did not achieve pregnancy, 32% experienced a third ectopic gestation, and 26% had at least one intrauterine pregnancy (9). Of 24 patients who underwent total salpingectomy for a first ectopic pregnancy and linear (or partial) salpingostomy for a second ectopic pregnancy in the opposite tube, those who attempted to conceive had an intrauterine pregnancy rate of 50% and a 27.8% incidence of third ectopic gestation (10). An estimated 50% of patients with a previous ectopic pregnancy will require treatment for subsequent fertility problems (11). These women should be advised to seek active surveillance for ectopic gestation during the next pregnancy.

Infertility Therapy

Controlled ovarian hyperstimulation, with and without assisted reproductive technology, has recently been evaluated as a risk factor for EP. Indeed, this complication was reported as early as 1976 by Steptoe and Edwards, whose first pregnancy achieved by in vitro fertilization (IVF) was an ectopic gestation (12). The incidence of EP after IVF currently ranges from 4% to 11% and is presumed to be secondary to the preselection of patients with tubal disease for IVF (13,14).

A study involving a small series of patients undergoing only ovulation induction revealed that this type of infertility therapy was also associated with an increased risk of EP, probably due to the effect of high estradiol levels on tubal egg transport (15). In addition, EP has been observed in unstimulated IVF cycles when patients did not receive any medication for ovarian stimulation (16). In this case, EP may occur as a result of transfer of embryos high into the interstitium.

One major concern is the higher incidence of heterotopic pregnancy—that is, the concurrent intrauterine and ectopic gestation following IVF. Historically, the incidence of heterotopic pregnancy was reported as ranging from 1 per 15,000 to 1 per 30,000 pregnancies (17). With the advent of ovulation induction agents and the attendant rise in dizygotic twinning and ectopic pregnancies, this incidence has increased to 1 per 4000 pregnancies in the general population and to 1 per 100 pregnancies following IVF (18). This potentially fatal condition can easily be overlooked once a gestational sac becomes evident in the uterine cavity. In the presence of controlled ovarian hyperstimulation, ultrasonographic confirmation of a gestational sac does not exclude a concomitant ectopic pregnancy.

Other Factors

The effect of infertility on EP rates is difficult to assess because of the known and unknown multifactorial components responsible for infertility. Nevertheless, the net effect is that each of several patient characteristics and behaviors may contribute to an increased risk of EP. The relative contribution of each for risk becomes evident through meta-analysis of multiple studies meeting specific inclusionary criteria. A recent meta-analysis of the current literature on risk factors and EP has been reported (19). Of the 211 manuscripts identified by Medline, only 36 manuscripts met the following criteria:

1. Case-control or cohort studies.
2. In cohort studies,
    a. EP was confirmed by operative or histopathology report.
    b. Women exposed to risk factors were compared to nonexposed controls.
3. Controls were defined as pregnant or nonpregnant.

The case-control analysis of 27 studies that included pregnant controls generally found that those factors affecting tubal integrity affected EP risk as well. The odds:ratio (OR) is considered significant if it is greater than 1, yet within the 95% confidence interval (CI) (Fig. 1.7). The common OR for chlamydia IgG exceeds 1:32; the ORs for gonorrhea, PID, previous

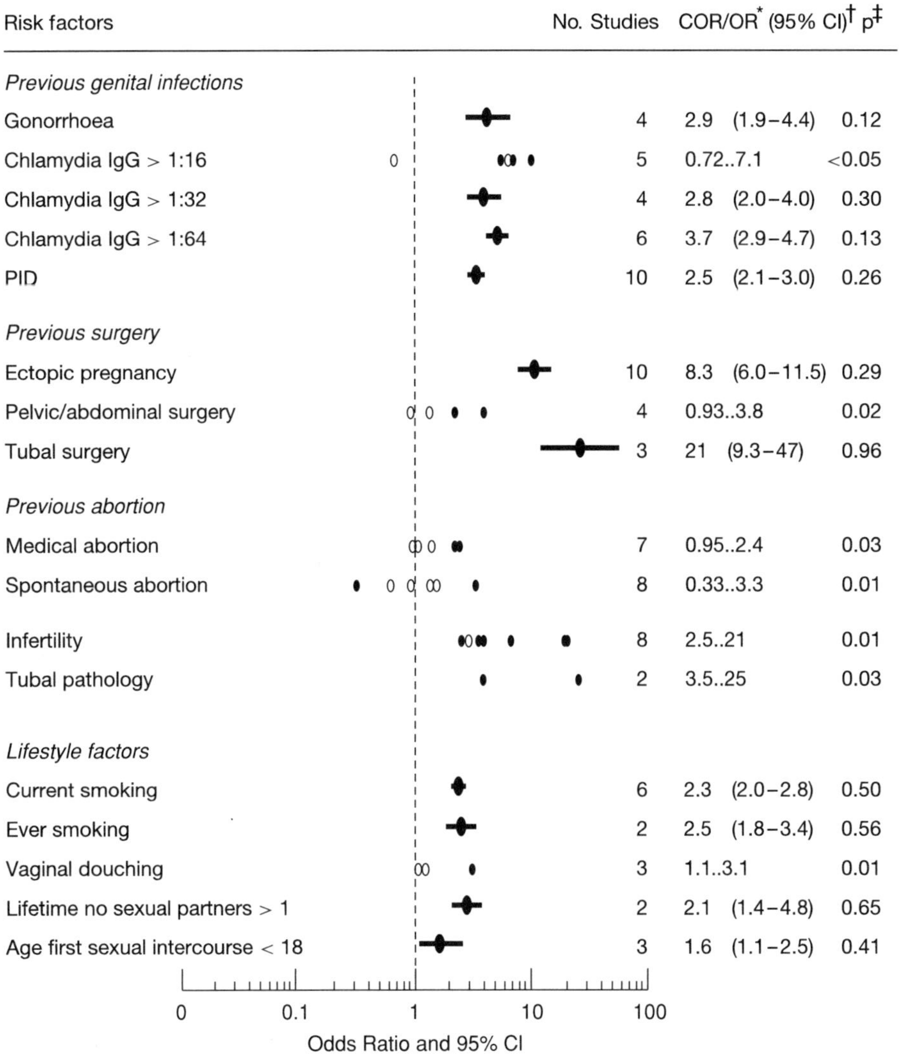
Risk factors
No. Studies
COR/OR* (95% CI)† p‡
Previous genital infections
Gonorrhoea 4 2.9 (1.9–4.4) 0.12
Chlamydia IgG > 1:16 5 0.72..7.1 <0.05
Chlamydia IgG > 1:32 4 2.8 (2.0–4.0) 0.30
Chlamydia IgG > 1:64 6 3.7 (2.9–4.7) 0.13
PID 10 2.5 (2.1–3.0) 0.26
Previous surgery
Ectopic pregnancy 10 8.3 (6.0–11.5) 0.29
Pelvic/abdominal surgery 4 0.93..3.8 0.02
Tubal surgery 3 21 (9.3–47) 0.96
Previous abortion
Medical abortion 7 0.95..2.4 0.03
Spontaneous abortion 8 0.33..3.3 0.01
Infertility 8 2.5..21 0.01
Tubal pathology 2 3.5..25 0.03
Lifestyle factors
Current smoking 6 2.3 (2.0–2.8) 0.50
Ever smoking 2 2.5 (1.8–3.4) 0.56
Vaginal douching 3 1.1..3.1 0.01
Lifetime no sexual partners > 1 2 2.1 (1.4–4.8) 0.65
Age first sexual intercourse < 18 3 1.6 (1.1–2.5) 0.41
0
0.1
1
10
100
Odds Ratio and 95% CI

FIG. 1.7.

Meta-analysis of case-control studies with pregnant controls. * = Common OR/range of ORs; † = 95% CI; ‡ = Breslow-Day test statistic on homogeneity; ● = common OR; • = significant OR of a single study; o = not significant OR of a single study; —— = 95% CI. (Reprinted with permission from Ankum WM, Mol BW, Van der Veen F, Bossuyt PM. Risk factors for ectopic pregnancy: a meta-analysis. Fertil Steril 1996;65:1093–1099.)

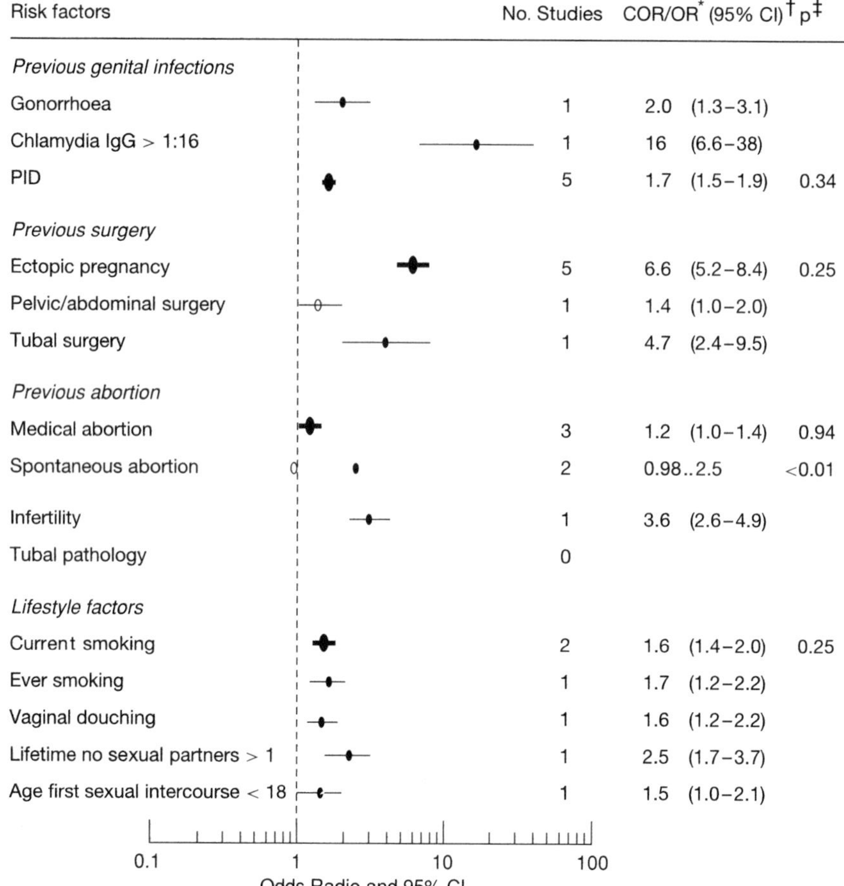

FIG. 1.8.

Meta-analysis of case-control studies with nonpregnant controls. ∗ = Common OR/range of ORs; † = 95% CI; ‡ = Breslow-Day test statistic on homogeneity; ● = common OR; • = significant OR of a single study; o = not significant OR of a single study; —— = 95% CI. (Reprinted with permission from Ankum WM, Mol BW, Van der Veen F, Bossuyt PM. Risk factors for ectopic pregnancy: a meta-analysis. Fertil Steril 1996;65:1093–1099.)

EP, and tubal surgery range from 2.1 for PID to 21 for prior tubal surgery. The common ORs for lifestyle factors such as current or ever smoking, more than one sexual partner over a lifetime, and first intercourse before age 18 range from 1.6 to 2.5. Risk factors that were not considered in all studies provide additional information. For infertility and tubal pathology, most individual ORs should show significant association with EP risk. Conversely, most ORs for events such as pelvic or abdominal surgery, medical or spontaneous abortion, and vaginal douching are less than 1.

The findings in case-control studies that used nonpregnant controls were in concordance with those reported for the case-control studies involving pregnant controls (Fig. 1.8). The authors explained the consistently lower common ORs found with the nonpregnant controls as relating to the difference in the probability of these patients having the risk factors responsible for EP; these risk factors are the same as the risk factors for infertility. For example, the common OR of EP for tubal surgery is found to be 21 in studies using pregnant controls but 4.7 in studies using nonpregnant controls. The significantly higher OR for the pregnant-control studies reflects the adverse effect of tubal surgery on fertility.

The results of the nine cohort studies were also in accordance with the case-control studies (Fig. 1.9).

As a whole, this meta-analysis provides useful information to the clinician in triaging those patients at risk and providing appropriate active surveillance of patients for pregnancy location (Table 1.1). Although PID appears to be less predictive of EP, its sequela of tubal pathology nevertheless makes this disease a strong risk factor.

Risk factors	No. Studies	COR/OR[*]	(95% CI)[†]	p[‡]
Pelvic and/or abdominal surgery	2	1.5	1.1–2.6	0.90
In utero DES-exposure	5	5.6	2.4–13	0.49
PID	1	5.7	2.5–13	NA
Medical abortion	1	1.2	0.78–1.2	NA
Infertility	1	2.0	1.2–3.4	NA

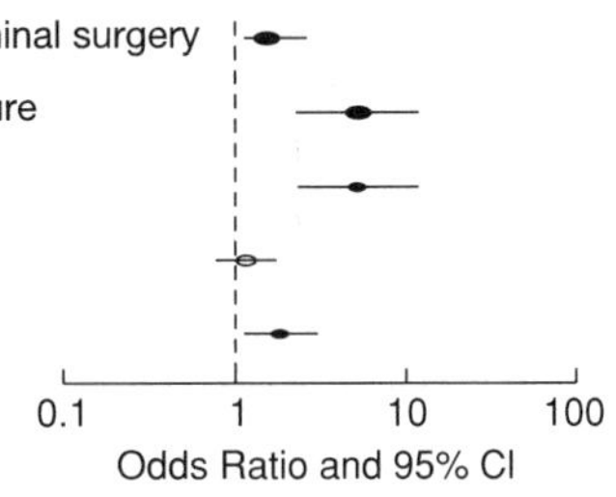

Odds Ratio and 95% CI (scale: 0.1, 1, 10, 100)

FIG. 1.9.

Meta-analysis of cohort studies. $*$ = Common OR/range of ORs; $\dagger$ = 95% CI; $\ddagger$ = Breslow-Day test statistic on homogeneity; ● = common OR; • = significant OR of a single study; o = not significant OR of a single study; —— = 95% CI. (Reprinted with permission from Ankum WM, Mol BW, Van der Veen F, Bossuyt PM. Risk factors for ectopic pregnancy: a meta-analysis. Fertil Steril 1996;65:1093–1099.)

TABLE 1.1

Strong and Moderate Risk Factors for Ectopic Pregnancy

RISK	RISK FACTOR
Strong	Previous ectopic pregnancy
	Previous tubal surgery
	Tubal pathology
	DES exposure in utero
Moderate	PID
	Infertility
	Lifetime number of sexual partners >1
	Current smoking

CONCLUSION

The consistent increase in treated EP noted over the period 1970–1992, in both hospital and ambulatory settings, may be due to several factors, including a heightened physician awareness, the availability of more sensitive diagnostic tools, and a true increase in the previously discussed risk factors for EP. Other factors that may increase a woman's risk of EP include maternal cigarette smoking, current use of an intrauterine device (IUD), and taking a progestogen-only contraceptive (OC) (19).

REFERENCES

1. CDC. Ectopic pregnancy in the United States, 1970–1983. CDC surveillance summaries, August 1986. MMWR 1986;35:29SS–37SS.
2. CDC. Surveillance for ectopic pregnancy, United States, 1970–1989. CDC surveillance summaries, December 1993. MMWR 1993;42:73–85.
3. Westrom L, Joesoef R, Reynolds G, Hadu A, Thompson SE. Pelvic inflammatory disease and fertility. Sex Trans Dis 1992;19:185–192.

4. Joesoef MR, Westrom L, Reynolds G, et al. Recurrence of ectopic pregnancy: the role of salpingitis. Am J Obstet Gynecol 1991;165:46–50.

5. Bernstine R, Kennedy WR, Waldron J. Acute pelvic inflammatory disease: a clinical follow-up. Int J Fertil 1987;32:229–232.

6. Marana R, Muzii L, Rizzim M, et al. Salpingoscopy in patients with contralateral ectopic pregnancy. Fertil Steril 1991;55:838–840.

7. Makinen JI, Salami TA, Mikkanen VP, Juhani-Koskinen EY. Encouraging rates of fertility after ectopic pregnancy. Int J Fertil 1989;34:46.

8. Nagamani M, London S, St. Amand P. Factors influencing fertility after ectopic pregnancy. Am J Obstet Gynecol 1984;149:533.

9. Clusen I, Frost L, Borlum KG. Reproductive outcome following two ectopic gestations: results after conservative surgery. Int J Fertil 1992;37:204–208.

10. Tulandi T. Reproductive performance of women after two tubal ectopic pregnancies. Fertil Steril 1988;50:164–166.

11. Bronson RA. Tubal pregnancy and infertility. Fertil Steril 1977;28:221.

12. Steptoe PC, Edwards RG. Reimplantation of a human embryo with a subsequent tubal pregnancy. Lancet 1976;1:880–882.

13. Yovich JL, Turner SR, Murphy AJ. Embryo transfer technique as a cause of ectopic pregnancies in vitro fertilization. Fertil Steril 1985;44:318–321.

14. Cohen J, Mayaux MJ, Guihjard-Moscato ML, Schwartz D. In vitro fertilization and embryo transfer: a collaborative study of 1163 pregnancies on the incidence and risk factors of ectopic pregnancies. Hum Reprod 1986;1:255–258.

15. Fernandez H, Coste J, Job-Spira N. Controlled ovarian hyperstimulation as a risk factor for ectopic pregnancy. Obstet Gynecol 1991;78:656–659.

16. Foulot H, Ranoux C, Dubuisson JB, et al. In vitro fertilization without ovarian stimulation: a simplified protocol applied in 80 cycles. Fertil Steril 1989;52:617–621.

17. DeVoe RW, Pratt JH. Simultaneous intra and extrauterine pregnancy. Am J Obstet Gynecol 1948;56:1119–1121.

18. Ory SJ. New options for diagnosis and treatment of ectopic pregnancy. JAMA 1992;267:534–537.

19. Ankum WM, Mol BWJ, Van der Veen F, Bossuyt PMM. Risk factors for ectopic pregnancy: a meta-analysis. Fertil Steril 1996;65:1093–1099.

2

Histopathology

Nilsa C. Ramirez

An ectopic pregnancy occurs when the developing blastocyst becomes implanted at a site other than the mucosa of the endometrial cavity. In more than 95% of cases, the site of implantation is the fallopian tube (Fig. 2.1). Ectopic pregnancies are also observed in other sites, including the ovary (Fig. 2.2), the abdominal cavity, the intramural or cornual portion (Fig. 2.3) of the fallopian tube (interstitial pregnancy), and the uterine cervix (1). Ectopic pregnancies located in the liver (2) and the spleen (3) have been reported as well. Tubal pregnancies appear to be more common in the right side (1,4–7) and, although infrequent, bilateral tubal pregnancies have also been identified (7,8).

Heterotopic pregnancies (simultaneous tubal and intrauterine pregnancies) are reported to occur in 1 of every 10,000 to 30,000 pregnancies (9,10). An increase in the incidence of heterotopic pregnancies has been observed in association with the use of techniques of assisted reproduction (in vitro fertilization, embryo transfer) and ovulation induction, especially if the patient suffers from tubal disease (11).

The fallopian tubes must offer the appropriate environment to effectively — and in a timely manner — transport the ovum, the spermatozoa, and, ultimately, the zygote. Their failure to function as intended can impair fertility, resulting in either infertility or an ectopic pregnancy.

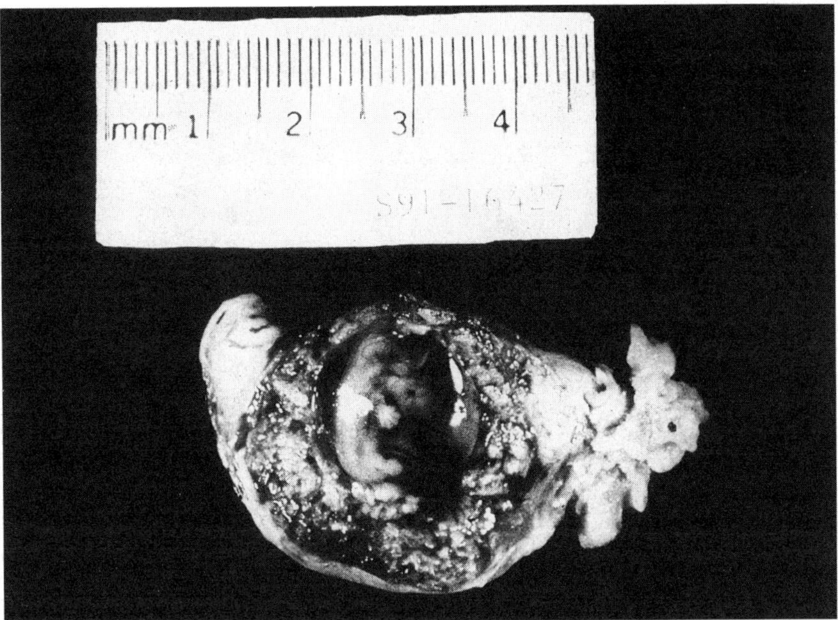

FIG. 2.1.

Tubal ectopic pregnancy. Note the intact gestational sac with an embryo.

Modifications of the fallopian tubes (of various etiologies) can cause both tubal and extratubal gestations.

THE FALLOPIAN TUBES IN ECTOPIC PREGNANCY

Embryology

The fallopian tubes are derivatives of the mullerian (or paramesonephric) ducts that form during the sixth week of embryonic life. During this stage of development, the lateral surface celomic epithelium of the paired urogenital ridges invaginates in several areas. Coalescence of those areas results in the formation of the paired mullerian ducts (12). As the female embryo develops, the ducts fuse by the end of the eighth gestational week (12); by the ninth gestational week, the fused ducts

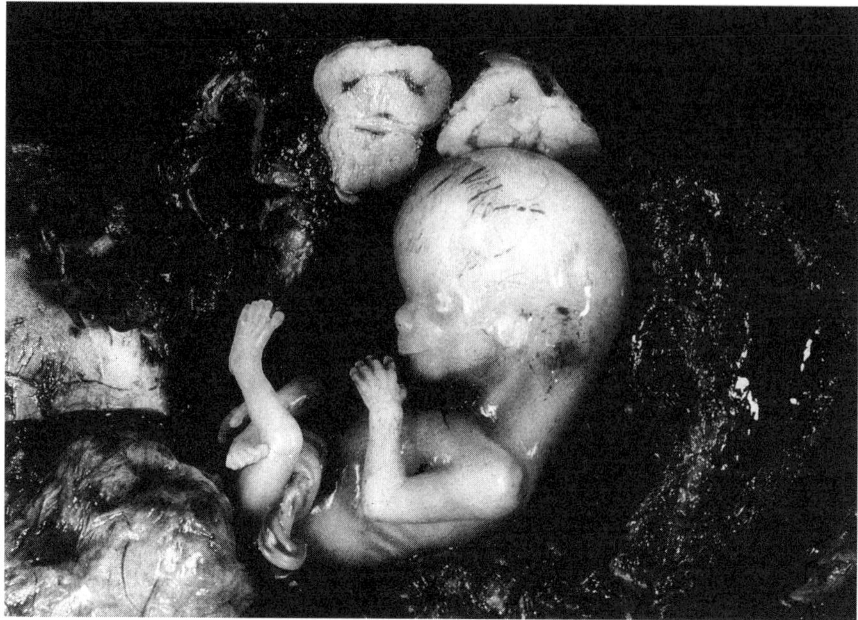

FIG. 2.2.

Ovarian pregnancy. The corpus luteum of pregnancy can be seen above the head of the fetus.

can be identified as the uterus. The uterine corpus differentiates into the endometrium, the myometrium, and the serosa by the nineteenth gestational week (13). Significant growth activity is noted in the fallopian tubes from approximately the sixteenth to the twentieth gestational week. The uterus, however, does not assume its adult form until the twenty-fourth gestational week (12).

The epithelium that lines the fallopian tubes exhibits variations in its characteristics during a woman's life in apparent response to the changing hormonal milieu. Ciliated cells, however, become apparent early during fetal development (14).

Anatomy and Histology

The extrauterine portion of the fully developed fallopian tube varies in length from 8.0 to 15.0 cm during a woman's reproductive years (15). Based on morphologic and anatomic variations, the fallopian tube can be divided into several sections or portions.

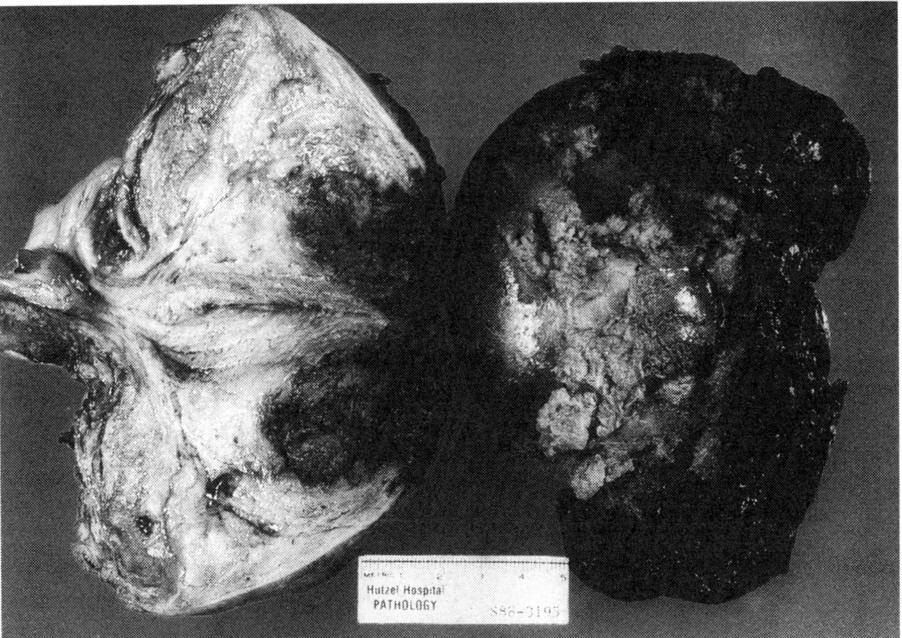

FIG. **2.3.**

Ruptured interstitial pregnancy. The placental implantation site involved the right uterine fundal area. The estimated gestational age of the fetus was between 16 and 17 weeks.

The proximal portion of the tube, known as the intramural or interstitial portion, lies within the myometrium. It varies in length from 1.0 to 3.5 cm and in luminal diameter from 2.0 to 4.0 mm (15).

The next portion, the isthmus, varies in length from 2.0 to 3.0 cm and in luminal diameter from less than 1.0 mm to as large as 2.0 mm (15). Approximately 10% to 15% of all tubal pregnancies occur in the isthmus (1) and, according to some workers, as many as 95% of them rupture (16).

The isthmus is followed by the ampulla, the longest portion of the tube and the area in which 75% to 80% of all tubal pregnancies occur (1). Approximately one-third of all ampullary pregnancies rupture (16). The ampulla varies in length from 5.0 to 8.0 cm and has a luminal diameter ranging from 1.0 to 2.0 mm (15).

In the more distal section of the tube, the funnel-shaped infundibulum, both the length of the tube and the luminal diameter average approximately 1.0 cm (15). The fimbriae originate at the infundibular area. At this point, the tube opens into the peritoneal cavity. Fimbrial gestations account for approximately 5% of all tubal pregnancies (1).

The wall of the fallopian tube has three major components: the serosa, the muscularis, and the mucosa. The serosa, which is the external coat of the tube, consists of flattened mesothelial cells resting on a thin sheath of vascularized connective tissue.

In the middle aspect of the tubal wall is the muscularis, characterized by two layers of smooth muscle: the thinner, outer longitudinal layer and the thicker, inner circular layer. An additional thin, inner longitudinal layer of smooth muscle, which becomes dispersed and scattered distally, extends from the intramural portion into the ampulla (15). Because interstitial connective tissue is present in the muscularis, layering of the muscle is poorly defined, especially in the outer longitudinal layer. Thicker layers of muscularis appear at the isthmic portion of the tube.

The mucosa rests on the muscularis and represents the innermost aspect of the tubal wall. Variations in its complexity throughout the length of the tube form the characteristic folds or plicae, the finger-like projections that occupy the tubal lumen. Approximately five broad and blunt plicae are usually seen at the intramural portion, although these plicae increase in number at the isthmus, where they become longer, slender and branch out. At the ampulla, however, plicae become noticeably more numerous and thinner and exhibit a more complex pattern of branching. The latter plical features can also be identified in the infundibular area. The fimbriae are finger-like extensions of the infundibular wall found at the distal end of the tube.

The tubal mucosa consists of a lamina propria characterized by well-vascularized loose connective tissue overlaid by epithelium. The connective tissue present in the lamina propria and in the submesothelial area can undergo a decidual reaction as a result of the hormonal alterations associated with an intrauterine or ectopic gestation. The epithelial lining of the tubal mucosa includes three types of columnar-shaped cells: ciliated, secretory, and intercalary (15).

The ciliated cells account for approximately 20% to 30% of the population (17). The synchronized movement of these cilia appears to play an important role in propelling the ovum toward the uterine cavity.

Additional factors (for example, tubal motility) may also contribute to ovum transport; patients with immotile cilia syndrome (Kartagener's syndrome), for example, are not infertile, although they do have impaired fertility. Each ciliated cell includes an oval to round nucleus, with a granular chromatin pattern and a small nucleolus. Controversy exists in the literature regarding the distribution of ciliated cells in the different tubal portions. Although some researchers claim that this type of cell is distributed equally throughout the tubal mucosa (18), others have found a difference in their distribution. Some studies, for instance, suggest that the ciliated cells appear to be more numerous at the apical aspects of the fimbrial and ampullary plicae (19) and relatively scarce at the intramural plicae (20).

Secretory cells account for 55% to 65% of the mucosal epithelial cells (17). Each secretory cell has an oval nucleus, with a small nucleolus and a chromatin pattern denser than that of the ciliated cell. These cells appear to play a crucial role in the formation of the luminal tubal fluid. This fluid has multiple components (21), including metabolic substrates, trypsin inhibitors, immunoglobulins (22), and electrolytes.

The third type of cell in the epithelium is the intercalary or peg cell (17). Such cells have dark staining nuclei and appear to represent a variant of the secretory cells (23).

Small numbers of lymphocytes — the majority of which belong to the T-cell suppressor/cytotoxic subgroup — appear to be a normal component of the tubal mucosa (24).

The epithelium of the fallopian tube undergoes changes associated with the hormonal alterations of the menstrual cycle (25). For example, increased estrogen levels appear to increase the activity of the secretory tubal epithelium and to positively affect the formation of cilia (26,27). In contrast, progesterone induces deciliation in the tube (28).

Tubal Pathology

Numerous studies have verified the association between a previous history of pelvic inflammatory disease (PID) and the development of ectopic pregnancies in 9% to 56% of patients (1,4–7,29). The tubal damage associated with previous bouts of PID results from acute and chronic inflammatory changes caused by a number of microorganisms, mainly bacteria. Other factors that appear to predispose a woman to developing ectopic pregnancy include a history of previous abdominal surgery (including tubal ligation), congenital anomalies of the uterus and/or fallopian tubes, intrinsic tubal pathology (of different etiologies), and hormonal abnormalities during the periovulatory and early luteal phases of the menstrual cycle. Some studies claim that a history of previous voluntary interruption of pregnancy predisposes women to the development of ectopic pregnancies; other investigations, however, have found no significant association between the two (7,30–32). In regard to intrauterine contraceptive devices, recent studies have failed to link their use with the subsequent development of ectopic pregnancies (7). Likewise, tubal endometriosis does not appear to be a significant predisposing factor (7).

A common denominator among the conditions associated with the development of tubal pregnancies appears to be the presence of some degree of tubal pathology. This pathology may range from significant anomalies (for example, hydrosalpinx) to alterations in the distribution of tubal epithelium (for example, changes associated with fluctuations in estrogen levels). Many patients have a combination of different pathologic conditions (7). In clinico-pathologic studies, some degree of tubal pathology is associated with ectopic pregnancies in as many as 90% of cases (7,33).

Although the exact cause of ectopic pregnancies remains unknown, the most common pathologic condition observed in the setting of a tubal gestation is chronic salpingitis. Reports linking the concomitant presence of chronic salpingitis and tubal pregnancy vary from 23% of all cases of ectopic pregnancy in a study by Breen et al (1) to 95.5% of all cases in a study by Dubuisson et al (33). Chronic salpingitis results from the resolution of an acute inflammatory process.

The risk of developing an ectopic pregnancy increases sevenfold following the development of acute salpingitis (34). The most common causative organism appears to be *Neisseria gonorrhoea*, although polymicrobial infections with organisms like *Chlamydia trachomatis* and *Escherichia coli*, as well as anaerobic bacteria, can also cause acute salpingitis (35,36). This condition can cause the fimbriae to adhere to each other and/or to the ovary.

If the fimbriated end becomes occluded, luminal pus may accumulate to form a pyosalpinx; if the ovary becomes involved, a tubo-ovarian abscess may develop. Resolution of a pyosalpinx may lead to tubal scarring and deformity or progress into a hydrosalpinx. A hydrosalpinx is characterized by a markedly dilated tube with a thin (often scarred) wall, few residual "normal" plicae, flattening of the residual epithelium, luminal straw-colored clear fluid, and (often) fibrous serosal adhesions.

Nearly 32% of the 571 histologically assessed cases of tubal pregnancies retrospectively identified in a five-year study performed in the author's institution showed evidence of hydrosalpinx (7). In the same study, hematosalpinx was associated with hydrosalpinx in 58% of the cases, significantly more than with any other single type of tubal damage recorded (7). This finding may reflect the thinning of the wall observed in the hydrosalpinx cases, which renders the tubal vasculature more susceptible to rupture and bleeding into an already-dilated lumen. The acute inflammatory process can cause fusion of the tubal plicae and, upon resolution, follicle-like (or gland-like) spaces may form, resulting in a pattern known as chronic follicular salpingitis (Fig. 2.4). It is believed that the developing blastocyst becomes trapped in one of the follicle-like spaces, where it eventually becomes implanted and subsequently develops.

The incidence of follicular salpingitis varies, with numerous studies having been conducted in this area. Nevertheless, this condition may occur in as many as 17.5% of all cases of histologically confirmed chronic salpingitis associated with tubal pregnancy (1). Organized fibrous serosal adhesions between tubal segments or between the tube and other pelvic organs can be seen as well. Chronic salpingitis, in general, is characterized by various degrees of plical attenuation and blunting. In addition, permeation of the tubal wall by plasma cells and lymphocytes is observed.

Salpingitis isthmica nodosa affects mainly the isthmus and, in approximately one-third of cases, the ampulla (37); grossly, it may present as nodularities in that area. Histologic evaluation reveals true tubal mucosal diverticuli that penetrate the wall at different levels and show concentric arrangement and hypertrophy of the tubal musculature around them, in a fashion similar to that of adenomyosis. This effect on the tubal musculature may explain why diverticuli that extend into the outer aspect of the wall may be detected grossly as tubal nodularities, sometimes reaching 2 mm in greatest dimension. The number of diverticuli is variable, inflammatory infiltrates are often absent, and no peridiverticular scarring

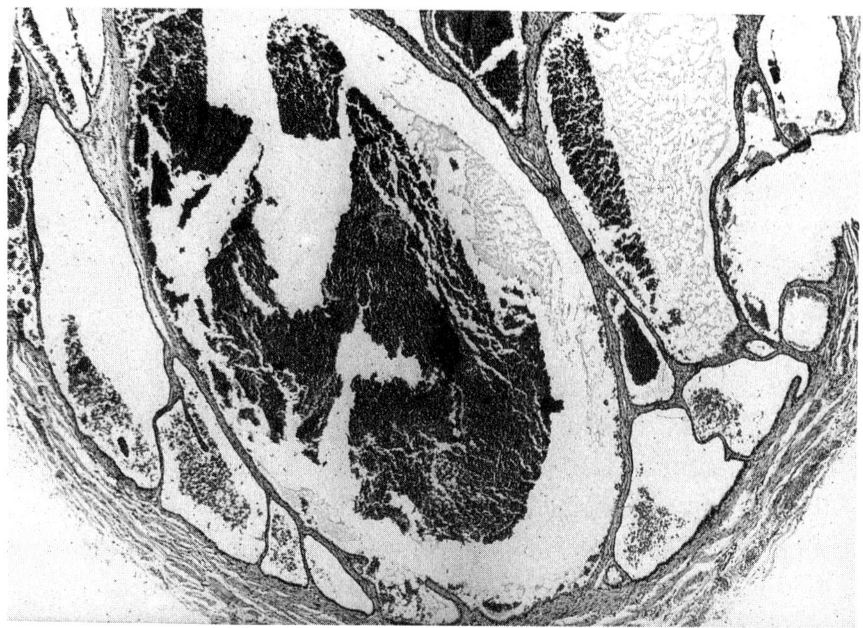

FIG. 2.4.

Chronic follicular salpingitis. Note the follicle-like spaces formed by the fusion of the plicae and the luminal hemorrhage.

occurs. Although salpingitis isthmica nodosa was originally thought to have an inflammatory origin, its true etiology remains unknown. Many investigators have suggested that a mechanism similar to that responsible for the development of adenomyosis may be at work.

The mostly bilateral lesion observed in salpingitis isthmica nodosa is associated with both infertility and ectopic pregnancies (37,38). The developing blastocyst may become implanted in one of the mucosal diverticuli and develop, eventually causing an ectopic gestation.

Salpingitis isthmica nodosa is found in 1% to 5% of all reproductive-age women but is uncommon before puberty and after menopause (38). In a study by Saracoglu et al (39), 10% of patients with tubal pregnancies had concomitant salpingitis isthmica nodosa, whereas the condition was detected in 7.4% of patients with infertility and tubal obstruction; only 0.2% of the control fallopian tubes had salpingitis isthmica nodosa.

In the five-year period in which the author's group studied ectopic pregnancies in our institution, 5% of all tubal pregnancies exhibited mucosal diverticuli. Interestingly, of the 29 (mainly right-side) interstitial ectopic pregnancies we identified, 18% were associated with mucosal diverticuli; none of these cases was associated with the gross nodularity usually seen in isthmic tubal diverticuli (40). The latter findings may reflect a propensity for mucosal diverticuli to occur in the intramural (cornual) portion of the fallopian tube. Patients identified through clinical investigative procedures as having mucosal diverticuli in those areas may represent a high-risk group for the development of interstitial pregnancy (40).

Patients with a history of previous ectopic pregnancy treated conservatively do not appear to have a significantly increased risk of a subsequent ectopic pregnancy in the same fallopian tube (7,41). Instead, the underlying pathology present in one or both tubes seems to be the determining factor in predisposing a patient to a recurrent tubal pregnancy (41).

Implantation and Development of Tubal Gestations

Upon gross examination, the tubal pregnancy varies depending on the status of the tube prior to the development of the implanted blastocyst. If the tube was not markedly distorted, an area (or areas) of mild dilatation may be observed, probably with blue discoloration secondary to bleeding. In a tube with hydrosalpinx, the dilatation may be marked, and the tube may resemble a cyst. Fibrous serosal adhesions may be present as well (Fig. 2.5).

Upon microscopic examination, the implantation site exhibits intermediate-type trophoblast involving blood vessels and the tubal wall in a fashion similar to the one observed in the uterus. Because the type of tissue that is able to undergo a decidual reaction is limited, it is not uncommon to see chorionic villi in direct contact with the tubal smooth muscle, in a manner identical to the implantation observed in a placenta accreta (Fig. 2.6).

In a recent study, Egarter et al (42) compared the proliferative activity of ectopic and intrauterine cytotrophoblasts using an immunocytochemical method and then correlated the results with the rising maternal levels of serum beta-hCG. Their findings indicated that tubal pregnancies develop at a slower rate than intrauterine pregnancies; in addition, they appear to exhibit variations in growth rate. In contrast, intrauterine gestations showed a faster rate of development, with all cases experiencing similar

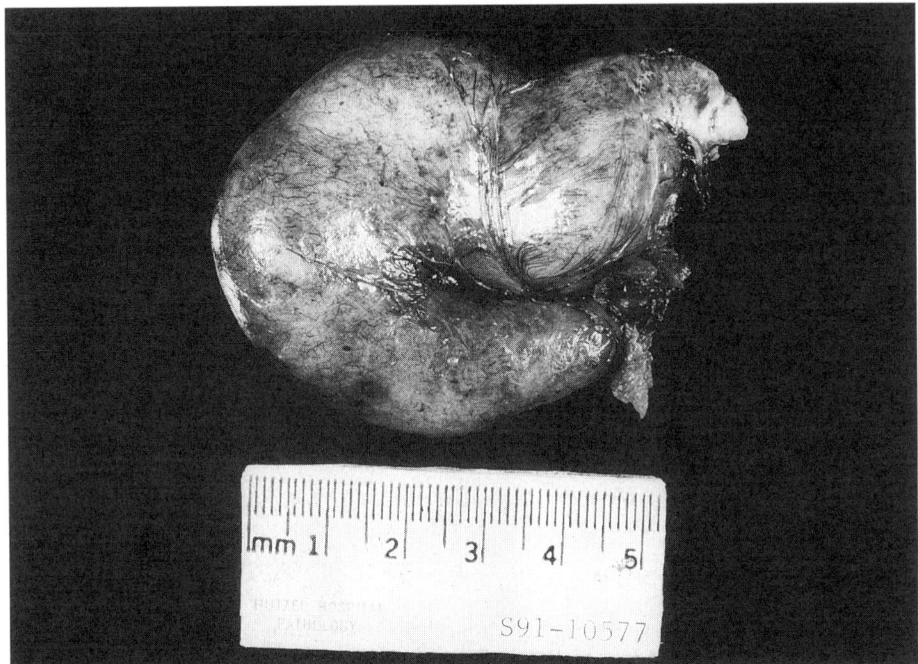

FIG. 2.5.

Tubal pregnancy associated with hydrosalpinx. Observe the distortion of the tube and numerous serosal adhesions.

growth rates. The rate of cytotrophoblastic development directly affected the increasing serum concentrations of beta-hCG (42).

In another study, Demir et al (43) compared the structure of intrauterine and ectopic (tubal) human chorionic villi using scanning and transmission electron microscopes. The ectopic chorionic villi exhibited architectural anomalies as well as decreased ramification and new villi formation (43). A delay in the development of the ectopic chorionic villi was noted after the fourth week of gestation as compared to the intrauterine chorionic villi (43). Also, other studies have shown that the tubal trophoblast is incapable of differentiating into chorion frondosum and chorion lavae (44).

The extension of the implantation site varies among cases, ranging from superficial involvement of the mucosal (plical) area to a totally transmural location. Tubal pregnancies rupture around the eighth week of gestation, and it appears that different factors may affect this process.

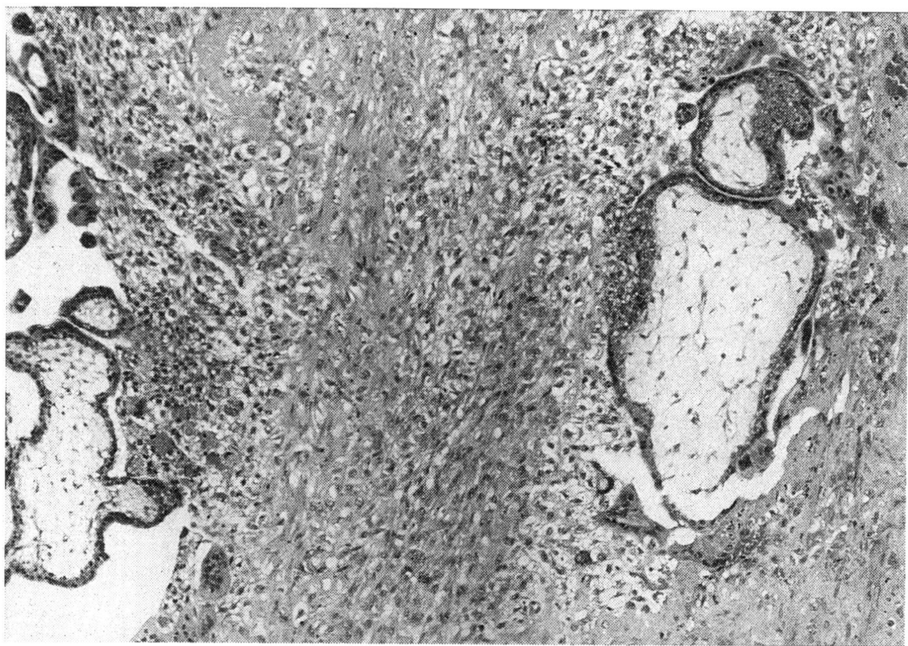

FIG. 2.6.

Implantation site. Chorionic villi can be seen in direct contact with the smooth muscle of the tubal wall, without intervening decidua (placenta accreta).

One important factor may be the increased luminal pressure generated by the developing gestation, which dilatates and weakens the wall. Another factor may involve the infiltrative nature of the anchoring trophoblast, which may weaken the wall and thereby render it susceptible to rupturing. Independent of the etiologic factors, it is not uncommon to find evidence of fresh hemorrhage, wall necrosis (sometimes accompanied by thinning), or transmural implantation of the gestation at the rupture site (7). Occasionally, early granulation tissue formation appears at the edges of the defect if sufficient time has elapsed between the event and the surgical removal of the tissue. Reactive mesothelial changes are commonly seen as well.

With the use of a vaginal probe and high-resolution ultrasound, embryos have been identified in approximately 23% of the tubal ectopic pregnancies (45). Fetal chromosomal anomalies, gross developmental anomalies (46,47), and gestational trophoblastic disease can be seen in association with ectopic pregnancy. Studies show that 2.5% of all gestational-associated choriocarcinomas develop following an ectopic pregnancy (48). The fact that the subsequent implantation of aborted viable tubal products of conception may be responsible for the development of extratubal ectopic gestations cannot be excluded.

Its clinical presentation can complicate the initial assessment of a "chronic" ectopic tubal pregnancy. This condition may present as an incidental finding discovered during evaluation for an unrelated condition or as a tubal mass, in the absence of detectable levels of beta-hCG. Microscopic examination usually reveals necrotic chorionic villi ("ghost" villi), sometimes with microcalcifications.

REFERENCES

1. Breen JL. A 21 year survey of 654 ectopic pregnancies. Am J Obstet Gynecol 1969;106:7:1004–1019.
2. Barbosa JA, de Freitas LA, Mota MA. Primary pregnancy of the liver. A case report. Pathol Res Pract 1991;187:2–3:329–331.
3. Yackel DB, Pantom ONM, Martin DJ, et al. Splenic pregnancy—case report. Obstet Gynecol 1988;71:471–473.
4. Bobrow ML, Bell HG. Ectopic pregnancy: a 16 year survey of 905 cases. Obstet Gynecol 1962;20:4:500–506.
5. Brenner FP, Roy S, Mischel DR. Ectopic pregnancy—a study of 300 consecutive surgically treated cases. JAMA 1980;243:673–676.
6. Green LK, Kott ML. Histopathologic findings in tubal ectopic pregnancy. Int J Gynecol Path 1986;8:255–262.
7. Ramirez NC, Lawrence WD, Ginsburg KA. Ectopic pregnancy: a 5-year recent study and literature review of the last 50 years. J Reprod Med 1996;41:733–740.
8. Adair CD, Benrubi GI, Sanchez-Ramos L, Rhatigan R. Bilateral tubal ectopic pregnancies after bilateral partial salpingectomy. A case report. J Reprod Med 1994;39:2:131–133.
9. Winer AE, Bergman WD, Fields C. Combined intra- and extrauterine pregnancy. Am J Obstet Gynecol 1957;74:170–178.
10. Levy G, Muller G, Pigaglio O. Grossesses intrauterine et extra-uterine simultanees. Rev Fr Gynecol Obstet 1987;82:729–732.

11. Dimitry ES, Subak-Sharpe R, Mills M, Margara R, Winston R. Nine cases of heterotopic pregnancies in 4 years of in vitro fertilization. Fertil Steril 1990;53:107–110.

12. Robboy SJ, Berhardt PF, Parmley T. Embryology of the female genital tract and disorders of abnormal sexual development. In: Blaustein's pathology of the female genital tract, 5th ed. New York: Springer-Verlag, 1995:8.

13. Silverberg SJ, Kurman RJ, eds. Embryology, histology and gross anatomy in tumors of the uterine corpus and gestational trophoblastic disease. Third series, atlas of tumor pathology, fascicle 3. Washington DC: Armed Forces Institute Of Pathology, 1992:1.

14. Patek E, Nilsson L. Scanning electron microscopic observations on the ciliogenesis of the infundibulum of the human fetal and adult fallopian tube epithelium. Fertil Steril 1973;24:819–831.

15. Woodruff JD, Pauerstein CJ. The fallopian tube. Structure, function, pathology, and management. Baltimore, MD: Williams and Wilkins, 1969:22–66.

16. Hu CY, Cheng FK. Tubal pregnancy: pathologic analysis of 300 cases. Chinese Med J 1958;76:6:517–528.

17. Dudkiewicks J. Quantitative and qualitative changes of epithelial cells of fallopian tubes in women according to the phase of the menstrual cycle. A cytologic study. Acta Cytol 1970;14:531–537.

18. Ferenczy A, Richart RM. Female reproductive system: dynamics of scan and transmission electron microscopy. New York: Wiley, 1974:212–253.

19. Patek E, Nilsson L, Johanisson E. Scanning electron microscopy study of the human fallopian tube. Report I. The proliferative and secretory stages. Fertil Steril 1972;23:459–465.

20. Wheeler JE. Blaustein's pathology of the female genital tract, 4th ed. New York: Springer-Verlag, 1994:529–561.

21. Mastroianni L Jr, Komins J. Capacitation, ovum maturation, fertilization and preimplantation development in the oviduct. Gynecol Invest 1975;6:226–233.

22. Kutteh WH, Hatch KD, Blackwell RE, et al. Secretory immune system of the female reproductive tract: I. Immunoglobulin and secretory component-containing cells. Obstet Gynecol 1988;71:56–60.

23. Novak E, Everett HS. Cyclical and other variations in the tubal epithelium. Am J Obstet Gynecol 1928;16:499–530.

24. Morris H, Emms H, Visser T, et al. Lymphoid tissue of the normal fallopian tube — a form of mucosal associated lymphoid tissue (MALT)? Int J Gynecol Pathol 1986;5:11–22.

25. Jansen RPS. Endocrine response in the fallopian tube. Endocrin Rev 1984;5:525–551.
26. Flickinger GL, Meuchler EK, Mikhail G. Estradiol receptor in the human fallopian tube. Fertil Steril 1974;25:900–903.
27. Gaddum-Rosse P, Rumery RE, Blandau RT, Thiersch JB. Studies on the mucosa of postmenopausal oviducts: surface appearance, ciliary activity, and the effect of estrogen treatment. Fertil Steril 1975;26:951–969.
28. Donnez J, Casanas-Roux F, Caprasse J, Ferin J, Thomas K. Cyclic changes in ciliation, cell height, and mitotic activity in human tubal epithelium during reproductive life. Fertil Steril 1985;43:554–559.
29. Riva HL, Kammeraad LA, Anderson PS. Ectopic pregnancy: a report of 132 cases and comments on the role of the culdoscope in diagnosis. Obstet Gynecol 1962;20:189–198.
30. Daling JR, Chow WS, Weiss NS, Metch BJ, Soderstrom R. Ectopic pregnancy in relation to previous induced abortion. JAMA 1985;253:1005–1008.
31. Burkman RT, Mason KJ, Gold EB. Ectopic pregnancy and prior induced abortion. Contraception 1988;37:1:21–27.
32. Chung CS, Smith RG, Steinhoff PG, Mi MP. Induced abortion and ectopic pregnancy in subsequent pregnancies. Am J Epidem 1982;115:6:879–887.
33. Dubuisson JB, Aubriot FX, Cardone V, Vacher-Lavenue MC. Tubal causes of ectopic pregnancy. Fertil Steril 1986;46:5:970–972.
34. Westrom L, Bengtsson L, Mardh P-A. Incidence, trends, and risks of ectopic pregnancy in a population of women. Br Med J 1981;282:15–18.
35. Chow AW, Malkasian KL, Marshall JR, Guze LB. The bacteriology of acute pelvic inflammatory disease. Am J Obstet Gynecol 1975;122:876–879.
36. Sweet RL. Anaerobic infections of the female genital tract. Am J Obstet Gynecol 1975;122:891–901.
37. Majmudar B, Henderson PH, Semple E. Salpingitis isthmica nodosa: a risk factor for tubal pregnancy. Obstet Gynecol 1986;62:73–78.
38. Honore LH. Salpingitis isthmica nodosa in female infertility and ectopic tubal pregnancy. Fertil Steril 1978;29:164–168.
39. Saracoglu FO, Mungan T, Tanzer F. Salpingitis isthmica nodosa in infertility and ectopic pregnancy. Gynecol Obstet Invest 1992;34:202–205.
40. Ramirez NC, Lawrence WD, Ginsburg KA. Extratubal ectopic pregnancy: a clinicopathological analysis of 41 cases. Lab Invest 1989;62:1:81A.
41. Stock RJ. Histopathology of fallopian tubes with recurrent tubal pregnancy. Obstet Gynecol 1990;75:1:9–14.
42. Egarter C, Husslein P. Proliferative activity of ectopic trophoblastic tissue. Hum Reprod 1995;10:9:2441–2444.

43. Demir R, Demir N, Ustunel I, Erbengi T, Trk I, Kauffman P. The fine structure of normal and ectopic (tubal) human placental villi as revealed by scanning and transmission electron microscope. Zentralblatt fur Pathologie 1995;140:6:427–442.

44. Randall S, Buckley CH, Fox H. Placentation in the fallopian tube. Int J Gynecol Pathol 1986;6:132–139.

45. Timor-Tritsch IE, Yen MN, Peisner DB, et al. The use of transvaginal ultrasonography in the diagnosis of ectopic pregnancy. Am J Obstet Gynecol 1989;161:157–161.

46. Poland BJ, Dill FJ, Styblo C. Embryonic development in ectopic human pregnancy. Teratology 1976;14:315–321.

47. Elias S, LeBeau M, Simpson JL, Martin AO. Chromosomal analysis of ectopic human conceptuses. Am J Obstet Gynecol 1981;141:698–703.

48. Lurain JR, Brewer JI, Torok EE, Halpern B. Gestational trophoblastic disease: treatment results at the Brewer Trophoblastic Disease Center. Obstet Gynecol 1982;60:354–360.

3

Diagnosis: hCG and Other Serum Markers

Edward C. Ditkoff
Mark V. Sauer

This chapter reviews how human chorionic gonadotropin (hCG) and other serum markers aid in diagnosing ectopic pregnancies and expedite the delivery of treatment to patients with this condition. First, it presents an overview of hCG. A description of normal and ectopic pregnancies follows, emphasizing surveillance monitoring using serum hCG levels. Other potential markers for discovering ectopic pregnancy, such as serum progesterone (P), 17-hydroxyprogesterone (17-OHP), estradiol (E_2), placental protein 14, relaxin, and plasma creatine kinase, are reviewed next. Finally, lesser-known tests, such as CA-125, human placental lactogen, active renin, alpha-amylase, SP1, alpha-fetoprotein (AFP) and prolactin, are discussed.

SERUM hCG

Human chorionic gonadotropin is a glycoprotein with a molecular weight of 36,700 daltons. Approximately 70% of the molecule is a polypeptide; the remaining 30% consists of carbohydrate. The carbohydrate portion is essential for the molecule's biologic activity.

Human chorionic gonadotropin has immunologic and biologic properties that are identical to those of other glycoproteins, such as LH, FSH, and TSH; all of these glycoproteins have common chains consisting of 92 amino acids. The β-subunit of hCG consists of 145 amino acids and is specific for hCG. Figure 3.1 illustrates the three-dimensional structure of the α and β chains of hCG. The α- and β-subunits have molecular weights of 14,500 and 22,200 daltons, respectively.

Since hCG was discovered by Hirose (1) and Ascheim and Zondek (2) nearly 75 years ago, its measurement has been the basis of pregnancy diagnosis. The first measurements of hCG focused on its biologic activity, which restricted detection to the intact, heterodimeric molecule. The advent of immunoassays in the 1960s (3) permitted not only quantification of the parent molecule, but also differential estimation of gonadotropin-free subunits and fragments.

Today, the isolation and characterization of an ever-expanding spectrum of hCG-related molecular forms in blood and urine have begun to enlarge the scope of clinical applications served by their measurement. Variations in the hCG molecule include the following: 1) those affecting sialic acid content (4−6) or carbohydrate structure and composition (7−9);

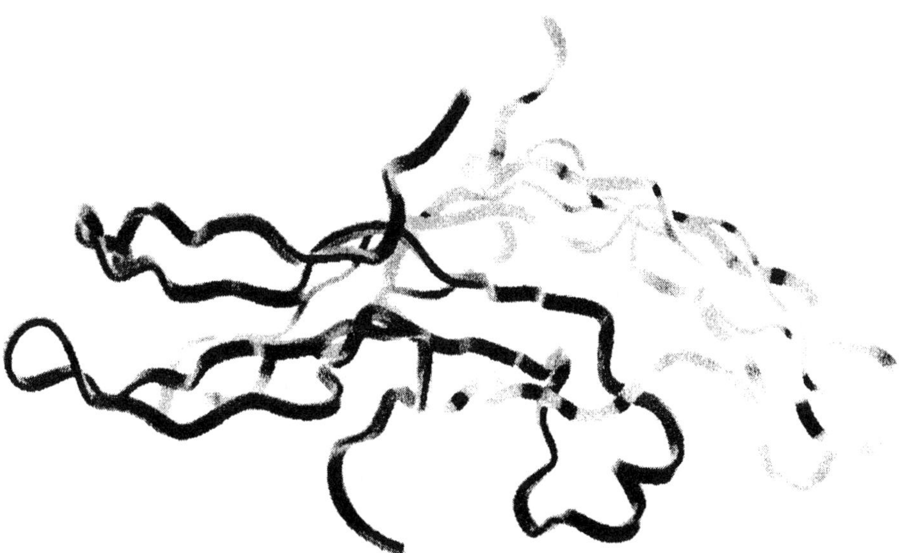

FIG. 3.1.

Ribbon diagram of hCG. The α-subunit is shown in black, and the β-subunit is shown in gray. (Courtesy of J. Lustbader, PhD, Columbia University.)

2) those influencing unusual free subunit concentrations in both pregnancy (10–13) and malignancy (14–17); and 3) those reflecting β-subunit peptide bond cleavages (18–21) and fragmentation (22,23).

Understanding the clearance rate of hCG is important for monitoring various pathologic situations, such as ectopic pregnancy. Figure 3.2 compares the disappearance of hCG, β-hCG, and α-hCG from the serum of normal male subjects after a single injection of the purified preparations (24). Table 3.1 indicates both the fast and slow component half-lives (in minutes) of hCG, β-hCG, and α-hCG (24).

The reference standard for hCG assumes primary importance when clinical judgments are based upon values measured by different laboratories.

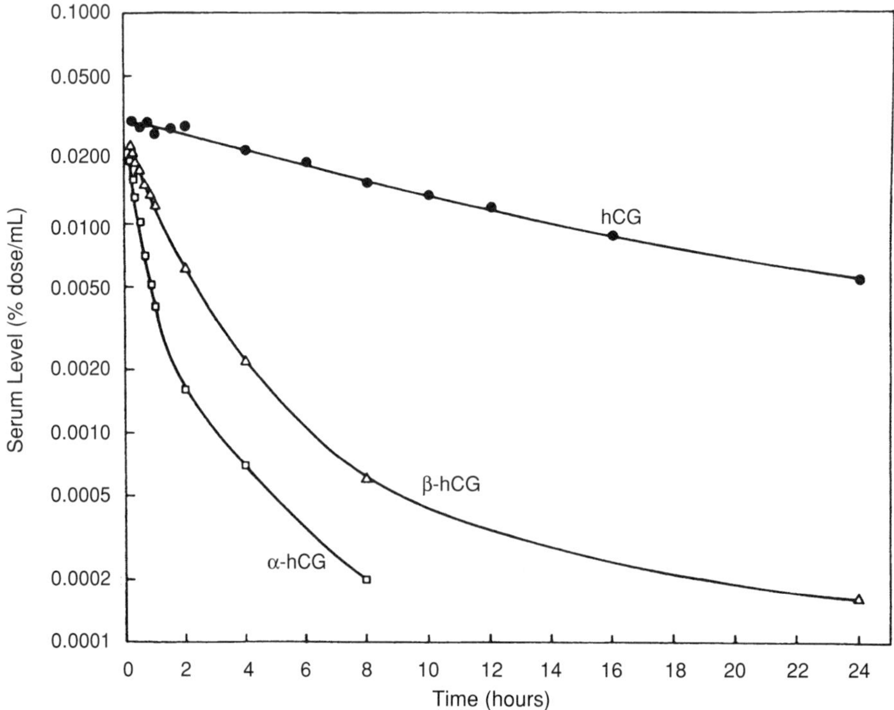

FIG. 3.2.

Comparison of the kinetics of disappearance of hCG, β-hCG, and α-hCG from serum of normal male subjects after a single injection of the purified preparations. Concentrations are expressed as a percent of the injected dose per milliliter. (Reprinted with permission from Segal SJ, ed. Chorionic gonadotropin. New York: Plenum, 1980:202.)

TABLE 3.1

Inital Apparent Volume of Distribution and the Half-Lives of
the Single and Slow Components Calculated from the Serum
Disappearance Curves of hCG and Its Subunits After Single
Intravenous Injection into Normal Men

PREPARATION	INITIAL VOLUME OF DISTRIBUTION (mL)	FAST COMPONENT HALF-LIFE (MIN)	SLOW COMPONENT HALF-LIFE (MIN)
hCG	3059 (±441)	415 (±72)	2390 (±415)
β-hCG	3601 (±974)	43 (±10)	239 (±109)
α-hCG	3158 (±441)	13.4 (±5.0)	94 (±75)

SOURCE: Reprinted with permission from Segal SJ, ed. Chorionic gonadotropin. New York:
Plenum, 1980:204.

The Second International Standard (2nd IS) hCG was established in 1964
by the World Health Organization (25). This standard was calibrated with
a variety of bioassays, and a pooled geometric mean was employed to
define the biologic potency of the 2nd IS hCG relative to the original
standard (1st IS hCG), which was established in 1938. The supply of
the 2nd IS hCG has since been exhausted. In 1974, large quantities of
highly purified hCG, both α-subunit and β-subunit, were donated to the
World Health Organization by the Center for Population Research and
the Reproduction Research Branch of the National Institute of Child
Health and Human Development (26).

Confusing matters even more, commercial hCG kits work with a
secondary standard, calibrated against either the 2nd IS or the International
Reference Preparation (IRP) hCG, rather than a primary standard. Because
several standards exist, it is important when using a set of reagents for
measuring hCG to take suitable steps to interpret the quantitative values
obtained by tests relative to each other. Most importantly, one should
attempt to work with the same lab using an identical assay and standard
when interpreting hCG values. This approach will allow correct clinical
judgments to be made when comparing results with respect to clearance
or doubling times.

hCG IN NORMAL PREGNANCY

Fertilization usually occurs within 24 hours of ovulation. The zygote rapidly undergoes mitotic subdivisions as it migrates toward the uterine cavity. This process takes approximately three to four days after fertilization. By the fifth day after fertilization, the morula or early blastocyst enters the uterine cavity (27). Implantation follows hatching, with the zygote becoming attached to the endometrium and invading through the superficial layer to gain access to the compact layer of endometrium (28). Normally, blastocysts become implanted along the posterior wall of the uterine fundus. As the blastocyst nestles into the endometrial stroma, it enlarges in mass and secretes hCG.

Detection of hCG in maternal blood has been reported as early as 6 days following ovulation. The first significant rise in serum hCG occurs 8 to 13 days after the estimated time of ovulation. Only after

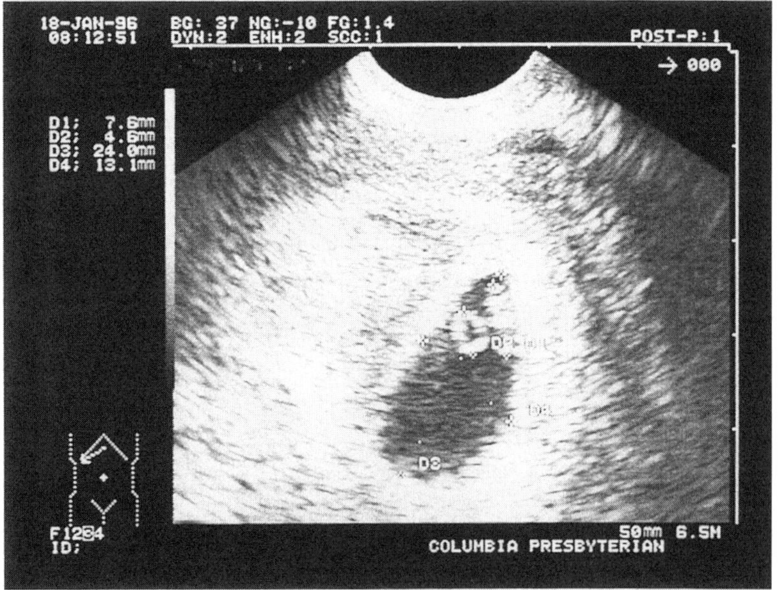

FIG. 3.3.

A single intrauterine pregnancy with cardiac activity seen at 5.5 weeks' gestational age. The gestational sac had a mean diameter of 22 mm with a yolk sac of 4 mm. One week earlier, a 10-mm gestational sac and 4-mm yolk sac were noted.

implantation and establishment of the uteroplacental circulation does hCG reach measurable levels in the maternal circulation.

At the time of the first missed menstrual period (two weeks postovulation), hCG levels are approximately 100 mIU/mL. At approximately three to four weeks postovulation, an intrauterine gestational sac becomes visible on ultrasound. Approximately one week later, cardiac activity may be seen. Correlation of transvaginal imaging to serum hCG levels varies according to the assay standard being used, but typically a gestational sac may be visible using a (5- or 7-mHz) probe with hCG levels of 1000 to 1500 mIU/mL (IRP). Cardiac activity becomes apparent with a level of approximately 5000 to 7500 mIU/mL (IRP) (Fig. 3.3).

During early normal pregnancy (three to six weeks postovulation), hCG levels rise exponentially, with a doubling time of approximately 3 days; levels peak at approximately eight to nine weeks (Fig. 3.4).

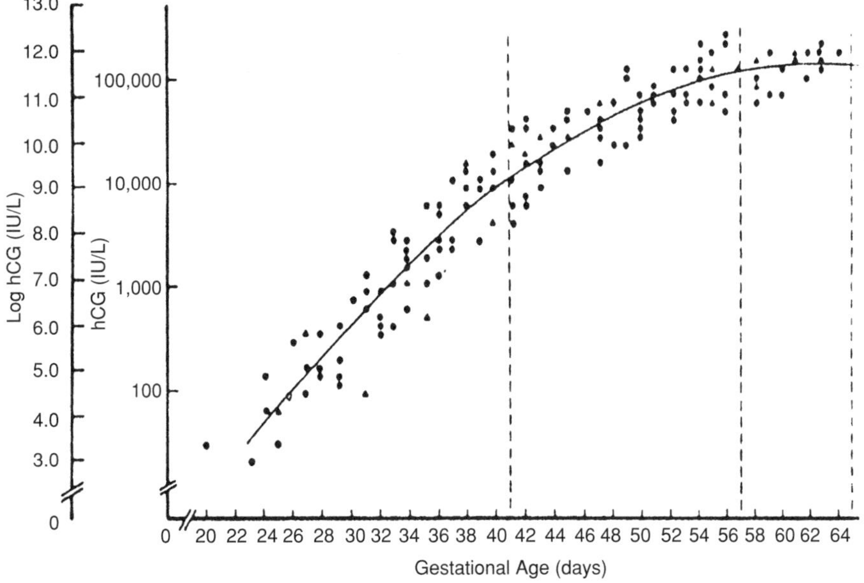

FIG. 3.4.

Normal increase in levels of serum β-hCG in early normal pregnancy. Depicted is a scattergram of log hCG plotted against gestational age, demonstating an increase in hCG levels until a plateau is reached at approximately nine weeks of pregnancy. (Reprinted with permission from Daya S. Human chorionic gonadotropin increase in normal early pregnancy. Am J Obstet Gynecol 1987;156:286–290.)

Although the doubling time of hCG has been assumed to be constant in early viable intrauterine pregnancies, it actually ranges between 1.4 and 3.5 days (29,30). The exponential rate of increase in serum hCG decreases with gestational age; hence the doubling time of hCG is not constant but rather becomes prolonged with increased gestational age. Doubling times could be 1.4 to 1.6 days from the first detection of hCG following ovulation until approximately 35 days after the onset of the last menses. They increase to 2.0 to 2.7 days, however, by days 35 to 42 after the last menses.

EXTRAUTERINE PREGNANCY

The principles underlying diagnosis and evaluation of early normal pregnancies using serum hCG allow the detection of an ectopic pregnancy by exclusion. In the first six weeks of gestation, serum hCG values are less than 6500 mIU/mL (IRP) and cannot be easily imaged. If the hCG level fails to rise at least 66% every two days or does not double more frequently than every three days, however, the pregnancy is considered abnormal. Ectopic pregnancies commonly demonstrate a slower-than-normal rate of increase. The clinical utility of a single quantitative hCG is limited, because one-third to one-half of all women presenting with ectopic gestations are uncertain of their last menstrual period. Nevertheless, when the level exceeds 1500 mIU/mL, ultrasound may be used in conjunction with a single value to discover a normal or abnormal gestation (Fig. 3.5).

Serial serum hCG measurements offer the greatest benefits in clinically stable patients. A single value for discriminating ectopic gestations requires ultrasound visualization of normal early pregnancy using landmarks as discussed previously. Thus hCG can be used to assess pregnancy viability, signal the optimal time to perform an ultrasound, and document the effectiveness of a diagnostic curettage (31).

Serial serum hCG measurements may also prove helpful in monitoring the treatment of an ectopic pregnancy, because persistent trophoblastic tissue secretes hCG. For example, during salpingectomy or salpingostomy, a rapid clearance in hCG would be expected to follow a complete excision of trophoblastic tissue. Initially, a decrease in hCG should occur, followed

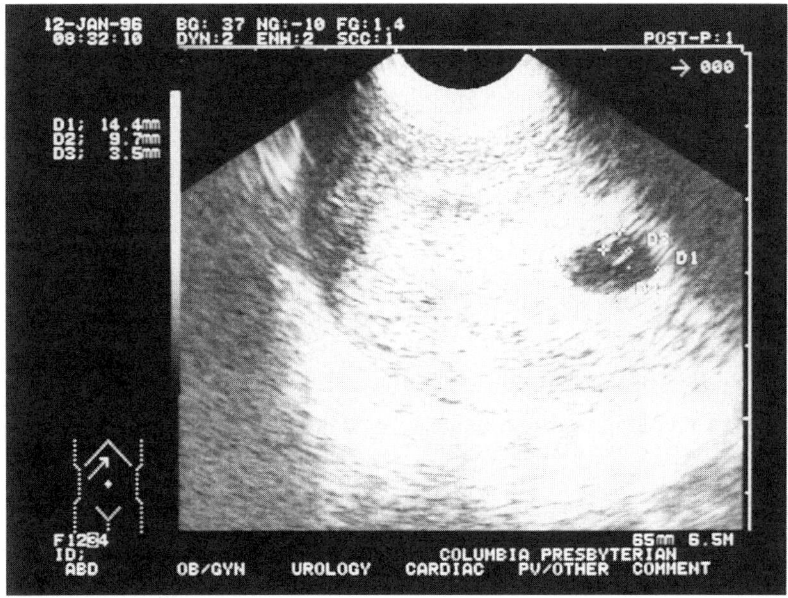

FIG. 3.5.

An early single intrauterine pregnancy is evident with a single β-hCG level of 2200 mIU/mL at five weeks' gestational age.

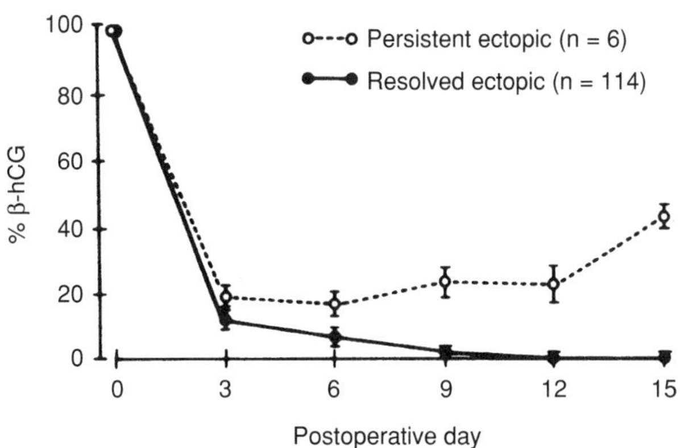

FIG. 3.6.

Serum β-hCG patterns in persistent and resolved ectopic gestations after salpingostomy is performed. (Reprinted with permission from Vermesh M, et al. Fertil Steril 1988;50:584–588.)

by an increase if viable trophoblastic tissue remains following salpingostomy (32) (Fig. 3.6). Consequently, all ectopic pregnancies should be followed until hCG reaches an undetectable level, which typically occurs within two weeks of the procedure.

When ectopic pregnancy is treated by nonsurgical techniques, such as injection of methotrexate, obtaining serial hCG levels again is critical. Levels should be followed every three to five days until they are undetectable. Other serum markers, such as progesterone and 17-hydroxyprogesterone, which have much shorter half-lives (less than one hour), have been used to predict the disappearance of β-hCG levels, as hCG takes as long as one month to clear because of its long half-life (approximately 30 hours) (33,34).

SERUM PROGESTERONE

Serum progesterone levels indicate the viability of the corpus luteum. Serum progesterone concentrations are elevated and change little during the first 8 to 10 weeks of normal gestation (Fig. 3.7). As pregnancies fail, progesterone levels decrease (35).

Serum measurements may contribute to the diagnosis of ectopic pregnancy in several ways. As an inexpensive screening tool, they identify patients who need further testing. Values less than 5 ng/mL are indicative of an abnormal pregnancy. Furthermore, if values are greater than 25 ng/mL, ectopics are excluded with more than 97% confidence (31, 36–39). A single value less than 5 ng/mL enables diagnostic uterine evacuation to be performed for cases where ectopic pregnancy cannot otherwise be distinguished from spontaneous intrauterine abortion (35,39,40). If progesterone values are less than 25 ng/mL but greater than 5 ng/mL, viability is best established via serial ultrasound examinations (31).

Unfortunately, reassurance cannot be given when normal levels of progesterone occur (5 to 25 ng/mL), as many patients presenting with ectopic pregnancies have values in this range (41,42) (Fig. 3.8). Thus, the role of serum progesterone in the management of ectopic pregnancy remains somewhat undefined. Based upon current published studies, use

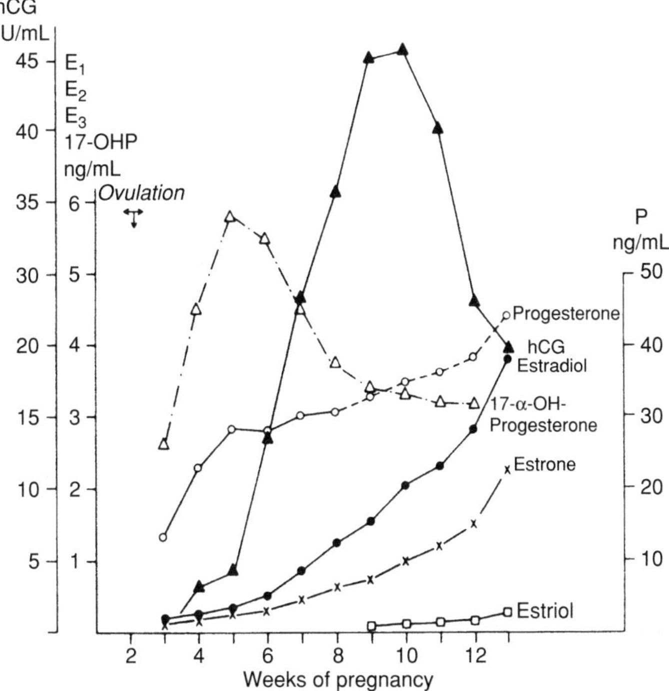

FIG. 3.7.

Mean plasma concentrations of progesterone (P), 17-hydroxyprogesterone (17-OHP), and estradiol (E_2) during the first 12 weeks of gestation, indicating the transition from steroid biosynthesis by the corpus luteum to that by the placenta. (Reprinted with permission from Tulchinsky D, Hobel CJ. Plasma human chorionic gonadotropin, estrone, estradiol, estriol, progesterone and 17α-hydroxyprogesterone in human pregnancy. III. Early normal pregnancy. Am J Obstet Gynecol 1973;117:884.)

of a single progesterone test appears to offer little advantage over serial measurements of β-hCG.

On the other hand, serum progesterone plays a significant role in monitoring of nonsurgically managed ectopic pregnancies using methotrexate. Progesterone levels fall to levels less than 1 ng/mL in successfully treated cases days to weeks in advance of β-hCG declines (32,33) (Fig. 3.9). This rapid decrease reflects the rapid clearance and short half-life of the steroid hormone (43). The fall in values results from

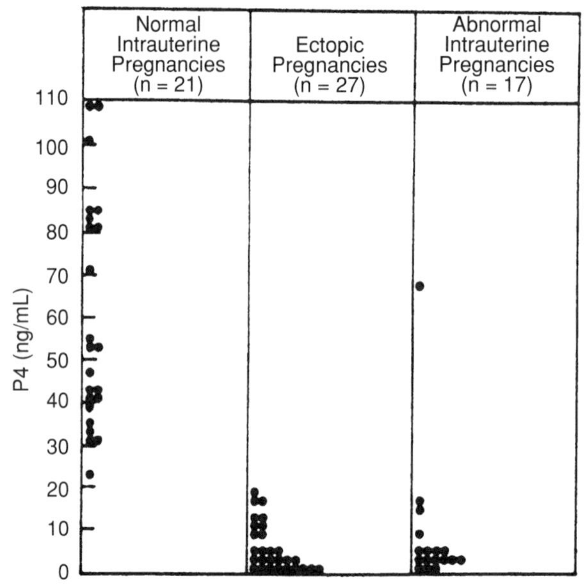

FIG. 3.8.

Progesterone levels obtained at the time of patient presentation for normal intrauterine pregnancies, ectopic pregnancies, or abnormal intrauterine pregnancies. All 27 patients with ectopic gestations produced progesterone levels of less than 20 ng/mL. (Reprinted with permission from Sauer MV, et al. Predictive value of a single serum pregnancy associated plasma protein-A or progesterone in the diagnosis of abnormal pregnancy. Hum Reprod 1989;4:331–334.)

decreased ovarian steroidogenesis, as methotrexate is toxic to the corpus luteum (33) and therefore destroys local trophoblastic production.

SERUM 17-HYDROXYPROGESTERONE

Serum 17-OHP levels reflect corpus luteum function more directly than serum progesterone levels, as the former hormone is derived solely from the corpus luteum, whereas progesterone originates from both the corpus luteum and the early placenta. During the first trimester in normal intrauterine pregnancies, the decline in corpus luteum function becomes

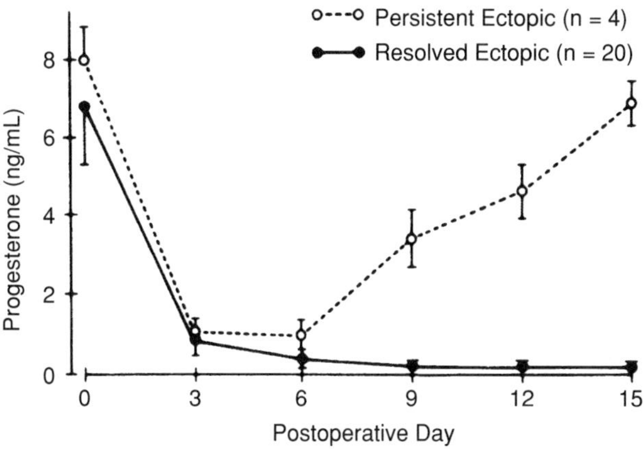

FIG. 3.9.

Serum progesterone patterns in persistent and resolved ectopic gestations after salpingostomy is performed. (Reprinted with permission from Vermesh M, et al. Persistent tubal ectopic gestation: patterns of circulating beta-human chorionic gonadotropin and progesterone, and management options. Fertil Steril 1988;50:584–588.)

evident when one compares serum 17-OHP and progesterone levels (44). As shown in Figure 3.7, serum E_2 and progesterone levels continue to rise progressively, whereas 17-OHP levels begin to decline at five weeks of gestation. Because ectopic pregnancies may be marked by abnormal corpus luteum function, 17-OHP might have utility as a marker. Clinical studies, however, have demonstrated that a single 17-OHP measurement is not diagnostic for ectopic gestations; in the studies, mean levels were similar to those of patients with spontaneous abortion. Furthermore, 17-OHP levels in ectopic pregnancies commonly overlap with the levels observed in normal intrauterine pregnancies (45).

Much like serum progesterone levels, 17-OHP levels may be used in nonsurgically managed ectopic pregnancies treated by methotrexate to predict the clinical response, because 17-OHP levels decrease prior to β-hCG levels (32,33) (Fig. 3.10). When treatment is successful, 17-OHP levels typically drop below 1.0 ng/mL, both initially and throughout the surveillance period, signaling resolution (33).

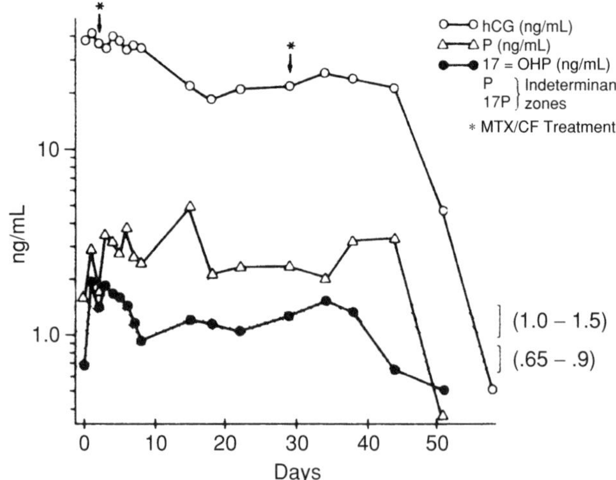

FIG. 3.10.

Levels of hCG, progesterone (P) and 17-hydroxyprogesterone (17-OHP) are demonstrated in a patient receiving two injections of methotrexate and citrovorum factor to effect resolution. hCG = human chorionic gonadotropin. P and 17-OHP levels are both lower and drop prior to hCG levels. (Reprinted with permission from Sauer MV, et al. Corpus luteum activity in tubal pregnancy. Obstet Gynecol 1988;71:667–670.)

SERUM ESTRADIOL

Similar to other steroid hormones, serum estradiol is derived from both the corpus luteum and the placenta. Kusco et al found no discriminatory cut-off value and considerable overlap in serum E_2 levels among patients with intrauterine and ectopic pregnancies (46). Similarly, Bustillo et al reported serum E_2 levels could not distinguish between IVF intrauterine and extra-uterine pregnancies or between viable and nonviable pregnancies (47).

SERUM PLACENTAL PROTEIN 14

Serum placental protein 14 (PP14) is a secretory endometrial protein. Romer et al found that low concentrations of serum PP14 were indicative of ectopic pregnancy (48) compared with spontaneous abortion or normal intrauterine pregnancies, especially between the fifth and seventh weeks of pregnancy. Ruge et al concluded that serum PP14 is regulated either by a control mechanism from the ovary or by paracrine secretion (49). These investigators also found that PP14 levels in patients with ectopic pregnancy are positively correlated with serum progesterone in women with ectopic pregnancy but not in women with normal intrauterine pregnancy (49). PP14 continues to be studied but remains of questionable clinical value.

SERUM RELAXIN

Relaxin was one of the first pregnancy hormones to be discovered. It was initially described more than 50 years ago (50). The corpus luteum of pregnancy serves as the most abundant source of relaxin. The physiologic importance of this hormone remains undetermined, however.

When Petersen et al studied variations in serum relaxin concentrations during pregnancy (51), they found that extrauterine pregnancies had levels of relaxin below the detection limit of the assay. In contrast, all normal pregnant women had measurable concentrations of relaxin higher than those with abnormal first-trimester pregnancies. Although relaxin has the potential to be a marker for ectopic pregnancy, its usefulness remains questionable at present and needs further evaluation.

PLASMA CREATINE KINASE

Recently, creatine kinase has been evaluated to see whether its measurement may have clinical value in the diagnosis of tubal pregnancies (52–54). Although the mean creatine kinase levels are higher in ectopic pregnancies than in other pregnancies studied, significant overlaps exist. Because serum creatine kinase has a sensitivity of 0.57 and a specificity of 0.67 for the diagnosis of ectopic pregnancy, it does not represent a reliable clinical marker (54).

OTHER TESTS

A variety of other serum proteins and hormones have been investigated for adjunctive testing, including SP1 (Schwangerschafts Protein One) (55), hPL (human placental lactogen) (56), prolactin (57), AFP (alpha-fetoprotein) (58), CA-125 (59,60) (Fig. 3.11), active renin (61), and alpha-amylase (62). Currently, these tests have only questionable value, because they tend to be time-consuming, difficult to measure, and expensive to run. Furthermore, as with other steroid hormones, overlap with other structured hormones makes them chemically problematic.

SUMMARY

With advances in technology, a greater efficiency in the early diagnosis of extrauterine pregnancies has been achieved. This advancement represents

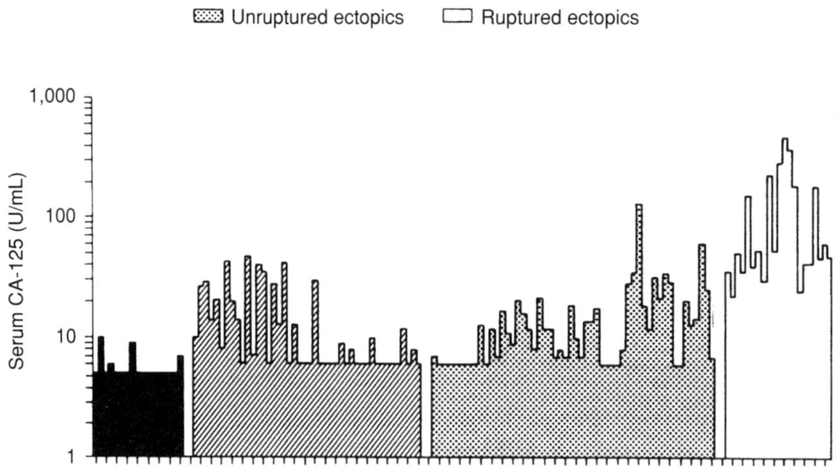

FIG. 3.11.

Depiction of raw serum CA-125 data for each of the 137 patients studied reveals a large overlap of values with various diagnoses. (Reprinted with permission from Sauer MV, et al. Serum cancer antigen 125 in ectopic pregnancy. Gynecol Obstet Invest 1989;27:164–165.)

a significant development, because much lower morbidity and mortality rates from extrauterine pregnancies are observed when diagnosis occurs prior to tubal rupture. To date, however, few serum markers have become available to aid in the diagnosis and no new markers appear to be superior to β-hCG. Nevertheless, adjunctive measures, such as vaginal ultrasound, when used with traditional serum β-hCG results have improved the management of patients with extrauterine pregnancies.

REFERENCES

1. Hirose T. Exogenous stimulation of corpus luteum formation in the rabbit; influence of extracts of human placenta, decidua, fetus, hydatid mole and corpus luteum on the rabbit gonad. J Jpn Geneol Soc 1920;16:1055.
2. Asheim S, Zondek B. Die Schwangerschaftdsdiagnose aus dem Harn durch Nachweis des Hypophysenvorderlappen-hormone. II. Pracktishe und theoretische Ergebnisse aus den harnuntersuchungen. Klin Wochenschr 1928;7: 1453–1457.
3. Wide L, Gemzell CA. An immunological pregnancy test. Acta Endocrinol (Copenh) 1960;35:261–267.
4. Imamura S, Armstrong EG, Birken S, Cole LA, Canfield RE. Detection of desialylated forms of human chorionic gonadotropin. Clin Chim Acta 1987;163:339–349.
5. Amr SM, Kasagi K, Ingbar SH. The role of subunit sialic acid in the thyrotropic and gonadotropic activities of human chorionic gonadotropin. Endocrinology 1987;121:160–166.
6. Cassels JW, Mann K, Blithe D, Nisula BC, Wehmann RE. Reduced metabolic clearance of acidic variants of human choriogonadotropin from patients with testicular cancer. Cancer 1989;64:2313–2318.
7. Blithe DL, Wehmann RE, Nisula BC. Carbohydrate composition of β-core. Endocrinology 1989;125:2267–2272.
8. Blithe DL. Carbohydrate composition of the α subunit of human choriogonadotropin (hCG α) and the free α molecules produced in pregnancy: most free α and some combined hCG α molecules are fucosylated. Endocrinology 1990;126:2788–2799.
9. Cole LA. Distribution of O-linked sugar units on hCG and its free α-subunit. Mol Cell Endocrinol 1987;50:45–57.

10. Cole LA. The O-linked oligosaccharide structures are strikingly different on pregnancy and choriocarcinoma hCG. J Clin Endocrinol Metab 1987;65:811–813.

11. Ozturk M, Brown N, Milunsky A, Wands J. Physiological studies of human chorionic gonadotropin; and free subunits in the amniotic fluid compartment compared to those in maternal serum. JH Clin Endocrinol Metab 1988;67:1117–1121.

12. Spencer K. Evaluation of an assay of the free β-subunit of choriogonadotropin and its potential value in screening for Down's syndrome. Clin Chem 1991;37:779–782.

13. Cole LA, Restrepo-Candelo H, Levy G, DeCherney A. HCG free β-subunit an early marker of outcome of in vitro fertilization clinical pregnancies. J Clin Endocrinol Metab 1987;64:1328–1330.

14. Alfthan H, Schroeder J, Frazer R, Koskimies A, Hallia H, Stenman U-H. Choriogonadotropin and its β-subunit separated by hydrophobic-interaction chromatography and quantified in serum during pregnancy by time-resolved immunofluorometric assay. Clin Chem 1988;34:1758–1762.

15. Macri JN, Kasturi RV, Krantz DA, Cook EJ, Moore ND, Young JA, Romer K, Laren JW. Maternal serum Down's syndrome screening: free β-protein is a more effective marker than human chorionic gonadotropin. Am J Obstet Gynecol 1990;163:1248–1253.

16. Ozturk M. Human chorionic gonadotropin, its free subunits, and gestational trophoblastic disease. J Repro Med 1991;36:21–26.

17. Iles RK, Lee CL, Olive RTD, Chard T. Composition of intact hormone and free subunits in the human chorionic gonadotropin-like material found in serum and urine of patients with carcinoma of the bladder. Clin Endocrinol (Oxf) 1990;32:355–364.

18. Huang S-C, Hsreh C-Y, Hwang J-L, Ouyang P-C, Chen H-C. Free α subunit of human chorionic gonadotropin in women with non-trophoblastic tumors. JH Formosan Med Assoc 1989;88:218–225.

19. Acevedo HF, Krichevsky A, Campbell-Acevedo EA, Gaylon JC, Buffo MJ, Hartsock BJ. Expression of membrane-associated human choriogonadotropin, its subunits and fragments by cultured human cancer cells. Cancer 1992;69:1829–1842.

20. Mann K, Siddle K. Evidence free β subunit secretion in so-called human chorionic gonadotropin-positive seminoma. Cancer 1988;62:2378–2382.

21. Cosgrove DE, Campain JA, Cox GS. Chorionic gonadotropin synthesis by human tumor cell lines: examination of subunit accumulation, steady-state-

levels of mRNA, and gene structure. Biochim Biophys Acta 1989;1007: 44–54.

22. Nishimura R, Ide K, Utsunomiya T, Kitajima T, Yuki Y, Mochizuki M. Fragmentation of the β-subunit of human chorionic gonadotropin produced by choriocarcinoma. Endocrinology 1988;123:420–425.

23. Puisieux A, Bellet D, Troalen F, Razafindratsita A, Lhomme C, Bohoun C, Bidart J-M. Occurrence of fragmentation of free and combined forms of the β-subunit of human chorionic gonadotropin. Endocrinology 1990;126: 687–694.

24. Nisula BC, Wehmann E. Distribution, metabolism, and excretion of human chorionic gonadotropin and its subunits in man. Chorionic Gonadotropin. New York: Plenum Press, 1980:199–212.

25. Bangham DR, Grab B. The second international standard for chorionic gonadotropin. Bull World Health Org 1964;31:111.

26. Storring PO, Gaines-Das RE, Bangham DR. International reference preparation of human chorionic gonadotropin for immunoassay: potency estimates in various bioassay and protein binding assay systems; and international reference preparations of the α and β subunits of human chorionic gonadotropin for immunoassay. J Endocrinol Metabol 1980;53:1090–1095.

27. Gasser RF. Embryology and fetology. In: Iffy L, Kaminetzky HA, eds. Principles and practice of obstetrics and perinatology, vol. 1. New York: John Wiley & Sons, 1981:127–181.

28. Hay DL. Discordant and variable production of human chorionic gonadotropin and its free α- and β-subunits in early pregnancy. J Clin Endocrinol Metabol 1985;61:1195–1200.

29. Pittaway DE, Reish RL, Wentz AC. Doubling times of human chorionic gonadotropin increase in early viable intrauterine pregnancies. Am J Obstet Gynecol 1985;152:299–302.

30. Aspillaga MO, Whittaker PG, Grey CE, Lind T. Endocrinologic events in early pregnancy failure. Am J Obstet Gynecol 1983;147:907–908.

31. Stovall TG, Ling FW, Carson SA, Buster JE. Serum progesterone and uterine curettage in differential diagnosis of ectopic pregnancy. Fertil Steril 1992;57:456–457.

32. Vermesh M, Silva PD, Sauer MV, Vargyas JM, Lobo RA. Persistent tubal ectopic gestation: patterns of circulating β-human chorionic gonadotropin and progesterone, and management options. Fertil Steril 1988;50:584–588.

33. Sauer MV, Gorrill J, Rodi A, Yeko TR, Buster JE. Corpus luteum activity in tubal pregnancy. Obstet Gynecol 1988;71:667–670.

34. Fylling P. Disappearance rate of progesterone following simultaneous removal of the corpus luteum and the foetoplacenta unit in women. Acta Endocrin 1970;65:284–292.
35. Kader N. Diagnosis and treatment of extrauterine pregnancies. New York: Raven Press, 1990:62–81.
36. Johnson MR, Riddle AF, Irvine R, Sharma V, Collins W, Nicholaides KH, Grudzinskas JG. Corpus luteum failure in ectopic pregnancy. Hum Reprod 1993;8:1491–1495.
37. Stovall TG, Ling FW, Carson SA, Buster JE. Nonsurgical diagnosis and treatment of tubal pregnancy. Fertil Steril 1990;54:537–539.
38. Stern JJ, VossF, Coulam CB. Early diagnosis of ectopic pregnancy using receiver-operator characteristic curves of serum progesterone concentrations. Hum Reprod 1993;8:775–779.
39. Ankum WM, Van der Veen F, Hamerlynck JV, Lammes FB. Laparoscopy: a dispensable tool in the diagnosis of early ectopic pregnancy? Hum Reprod 1993;8:1301–1306.
40. Ou CS. Laparoscopic management of ectopic pregnancy. J Reprod Med 1993;38:849–852.
41. Gelder MS, Boots LR, Younger JB. Use of a single random serum progesterone value as a diagnostic aid for ectopic pregnancy. Fertil Steril 1991;55:497–500.
42. Sauer MV, Sinosich MJ, Yeko TR, Vermesh M, Buster JE, Simon JA. Predictive value of a single serum pregnancy associated plasma protein-A or progesterone in the diagnosis of abnormal pregnancy. Hum Reprod 1989;4:331–334.
43. Yeko TR, Gorrill MJ, Hughes LH, Rodi IA, Buster JE, Sauer MV. Timely diagnosis of early ectopic pregnancy using a single blood progesterone measurement. Fertil Steril 1987;48:1048–1050.
44. Tulchinsky D, Hobel CJ. Plasma human chorionic gonadotropin, estrone, estradiol, estriol, progesterone and 17α-hydroxy progesterone in human pregnancy. III. Early normal pregnancy. Am J Obstet Gynecol 1973;117:884.
45. Choe JK, Check JH, Nowroozi K, Benveniste R, Barnea ER. Serum progesterone and 17-hydroxyprogesterone in the diagnosis of ectopic pregnancies and the value of progesterone replacement in intrauterine pregnancies when serum progesterone levels are low. Gynecol Obstet Invest 1992;34:133–138.
46. Kusco E, Vicdan K, Turhan NO, Oguz S, Zorlu G, Gokmen O. The hormonal profile in ectopic pregnancies. Materia Medica Polona 1993;25:149–152.

47. Bustillo M, Stern JJ, King D, Coulam CB. Serum progesterone and estradiol concentrations in the early diagnosis of ectopic pregnancy after in vitro fertilization-embryo transfer. Fertil Steril 1993;59:668−670.

48. Romer T, Straube W, Mesiel M, Wodrig W. Zum Wert der Plazentaprotein 14-Bestimmung im Serum zur Differentialdiagnostik der gestorten Fruhschwangerschaft. Geburtshilfe un Frauenheilkunde 1995;55:490−492.

49. Ruge S, Sorenson S, Vejtorp M, Vejerslev LO. The secretory endometrial protein, placental protein 14, in women with ectopic gestation. Fertil Steril 1992;57:102−106.

50. Siler-Khodr TM, Khodr GS. Production and activity of placental releasing hormones. In: Novy MJ, Resko JA, eds. Fetal endocrinology. New York: Academic Press, 1981:183−210.

51. Petersen LK, Vogel I, Agger AO, Westergaard J, Nil M, Uldbjerg N. Variations in serum relaxin (hRLX-2) concentrations during human pregnancy. Acta Obstet Gynecol Scand 1995;74:251−256.

52. Vandermolen DT, Borzelleca JF. Serum creatine kinase does not predict ectopic pregnancy. Fertil Steril 1996;65:916−921.

53. Korhonen J, Alfthan H, Stenman UH, Ylostalo P. Failure of creatine kinase to predict ectopic pregnancy. Fertil Steril 1996;65:922−924.

54. Duncan WC, Sweeting VM, Cawood P, Illingworth PJ. Measurement of creatine kinase activity and diagnosis of ectopic pregnancy. Br J Obstet Gynecol 1995;102:233−237.

55. Grudzinskas JG, Westergaard JG, Teisner B. Biochemical assessment of placental function: early pregnancy. Clin Obstet Gynecol 1986;13:553−569.

56. Carson SA, Stovall T, Umstot E, Andersen R, Ling F, Buster JE. Rising human chorionic somatomammotropin predicts ectopic pregnancy rupture following methotrexate chemotherapy. Fertil Steril 1989;51:593−597.

57. Biswas S, Rodeck CH. Plasma prolactin levels during pregnancy. Br J Obstet Gynaecol 1976;83:683−687.

58. Goldner TE, Lawson HW, Xia Z, Atrash HK. Surveillance of ectopic pregnancy: Unites States, 1970−1989. MMWR CDC Surveillance Summaries 1993;42:73−85.

59. Sauer MV, Vasilev SA, Campeau J, Vermesh M. Serum cancer antigen 125 in ectopic pregnancy. Gynecol Obstet Invest 1989;27:164−165.

60. Jacobs IJ, Fay TN, Yovich J, Stabile I, Frost C, Turner J, Oram DH, Grundzinskas JG. Serum levels of CA-125 during the first trimester of normal outcome, ectopic and anembryonic pregnancies. Hum Reprod 1990;5:116−122.

61. Meunier K, Mignot TM, Maria B, Guichard A, Zorn JR, Cedard L. Predictive value of the active renin assay for the diagnosis of ectopic pregnancy. Fertil Steril 1991;55:432–435.
62. Hannon ZJ, Guzick DS. Tubal pregnancy significance of serum and peritoneal fluid alpha amylase. Obstet Gynecol 1985;66:395–399.

4

Transvaginal and Doppler Sonography of Ectopic Pregnancy

Samuel C. Johnson

A significant rise in the rate of ectopic pregnancy has produced a heightened awareness of the disease (1–3). Ectopic pregnancy is clinically suspected approximately 10 times more often than it occurs, and 86% of patients who experience the classic triad of adnexal mass, abdominal pain, and vaginal bleeding do not have ectopic pregnancies (4,5). The clinical presentation of ectopic pregnancies varies according to the rate and degree of trophoblastic development, the integrity of the fallopian tube, and the site of ectopia.

A demonstrable decline in morbidity and mortality associated with ectopic pregnancy has largely resulted from earlier and more accurate diagnosis (2). Most important was the development of a sensitive and specific beta-hCG pregnancy test (6). Because a single beta-hCG value cannot distinguish between an intrauterine pregnancy (IUP) and an ectopic gestation, transvaginal ultrasound (TVUS) plays an important role in making this distinction (6,7). Improvements in overall diagnostic capability have likely contributed to the rising incidence of ectopic pregnancy, as many currently detectable ectopic pregnancies would have remained clinically silent with earlier diagnostic methods (8).

ULTRASOUND TECHNIQUE

Ultrasound is a highly operator-dependent modality, with its accuracy directly reflecting the expertise and experience of the examiner (9–11). Many technical, anatomic, and physiologic factors exist that can confuse the sonographic diagnosis of ectopic pregnancy (12). These pitfalls and errors of interpretation diminish with examiner experience, although they cannot be completely eliminated. As a result, adequate training and supervision are imperative for all personnel involved in performing diagnostic ultrasound, along with timely consultation and referral for difficult cases.

Transvaginal Ultrasound

The physical proximity of the vaginal ultrasound transducer provides dramatically higher spatial resolution of the pelvic viscera compared with transabdominal ultrasound (TAS) (13,14). The frequency of an ultrasound transducer is directly proportional to its axial resolution and inversely proportional to the depth penetration (15). TVUS probes generally fall in the range of 5 to 7 MHz, whereas TAS probes are rated at 3 MHz. The limited range of the TVUS probe compromises evaluation of structures situated high in the pelvis and prevents visualization of large pelvic masses in their entirety (9,15).

TVUS does offer the benefits of a short learning curve and shorter overall procedure time. This imaging technique is particularly advantageous in obese patients and retroverted uteri—both areas where TAS has pronounced limitations (16). TVUS is well tolerated by patients and largely preferred over TAS, as the latter requires maintaining a distended urinary bladder (17).

Despite the obvious advantages of TVUS, TAS should be considered a complementary—rather than an inferiorly competitive—procedure. Approximately 5% of ectopic pregnancies are located beyond the range of the TVUS transducer, and TAS must be employed to identify this subgroup (12).

Doppler Ultrasound

Doppler ultrasound adds physiologic information to the anatomic information provided by gray-scale images. The combination of a pulsed

Doppler beam with a gray-scale image (duplex scan) allows direct interrogation of identifiable vessels. Color Doppler offers the advantage of demonstrating smaller and more numerous vessels than can be seen on gray-scale images and provides a quicker, more sensitive, and more precise vascular examination (18).

Power Doppler is a modality that utilizes amplitude rather than the velocity parameters of blood flow. It offers greater sensitivity for detection of vascularity than does color Doppler (19).

Assessment of Doppler waveforms of small pelvic vessels relies on impedance rather than velocity measurements. Impedance (or resistance) is analyzed using one of two indices: the resistive index (R.I.) or the pulsatility index (P.I.). The R.I. equals the peak systolic minus end diastolic frequency, divided by the peak systolic frequency. The P.I. equals the peak systolic frequency minus end diastolic frequency, divided by the mean frequency shift of the cycle (20,21). Magnifying or zooming an area of interest, followed by adjustment of the Doppler parameters of pulse repetition frequency, Doppler gain, and filter, should be performed to augment Doppler sensitivity.

Scan Protocol for Ectopic Pregnancy

Table 4.1 details the scan protocol for ectopic pregnancy. Sonographic evaluation of the pelvis should be performed on clinically stable patients with suspected ectopic pregnancies. Unstable patients require immediate surgery, and an initial sonographic evaluation would create an inappropriate delay in definitive therapy.

Initially, TAS is performed, with a focus on regions not easily evaluated with TVUS. Bladder volume is not critical, as the high pelvic structures being assessed are located considerably above the level at which a bladder acoustic window is useful. Images are obtained in the right flank and Morrison's pouch in the right upper quadrant (RUQ), searching for significant hemoperitoneum. If the examination reveals a large amount of fluid, it should be terminated and the clinician notified. Prolonged sonographic attempts to identify and localize the actual ectopic gestation are typically futile and merely delay surgery, as extensive hemorrhage obscures pelvic anatomy. If the abdomen does not contain a large amount of fluid, the examination continues with TAS images of the uterus

TABLE 4.1

Scan Protocol for Ectopic Pregnancy

Transabdominal ultrasound
Image Morison's pouch and both flanks
Identify uterus and ovaries, if possible

Transvaginal ultrasound
Uterus: identify endometrium, cervix, and interstitial line
Ovary: visualize corpus luteum
Adnexa: survey for extraovarian adnexal masses, cul-de-sac fluid

Doppler
Uterus: interrogate endometrium for peritrophoblastic flow if no IUP seen
Ovary: color or power Doppler to identify corpus luteum
Adnexa: Doppler of any suspicious adnexal mass

and adnexae in an attempt to demonstrate an obvious IUP or ectopic pregnancy.

Before the TVUS exam begins, the patient should be asked to void. Even a moderate degree of bladder distention will lessen the angle of uterine anteversion, elevating the uterine body and fundus superiorly within the pelvis and positioning them beyond the range of the TVUS probe. The TVUS study is performed in a manner similar to a gynecologic pelvic exam. The patient is placed in the lithotomy position, with appropriate considerations being made for patient privacy. A disposable condom or sheath covers the gel-coated transducer. The subsequent deliberate examination of the uterus and adnexae relies on long- and short-axis views, with the operator creating permanent documentation of the findings. The small field of view in TVUS compromises anatomic orientation, and obvious landmarks may not be readily apparent, emphasizing the need for proper annotation of permanent images. Following the TVUS exam, the vaginal transducer is wiped clean and disinfected as recommended by the manufacturer.

COMBINED USE OF BETA-hCG AND TVUS

The volume of functioning trophoblastic tissue affects both the TVUS findings and the serum beta-hCG level, and correlating TVUS and serum beta-hCG results has aided in diagnosis of ectopic pregnancy (22). The concept of the discriminatory zone (DZ), which was developed by Kadar in 1981, describes the serum beta-hCG level at which an intrauterine gestational sac should always be identified on ultrasound (23). A beta-hCG level exceeding the DZ without a sonographically apparent IUP was once considered diagnostic of an ectopic pregnancy. Unfortunately, the DZ is not a uniform, constant, transferable value; instead, it must be individualized for specific institutions, ultrasound equipment, and beta-hCG reference standards (24). Both the technical capabilities of the ultrasound machine and the type of transducer employed will affect the ability to resolve an early intrauterine gestational sac. Use of the TVUS probe and further advances in ultrasound technology have seen a fall from Kadar's initial DZ of 6500 mIU/mL (IRP) to levels as low as 600 mIU/mL (IRP) (23,25–27).

The usefulness of the DZ concept is limited by the significant number of patients presenting with subdiscriminatory zone levels, which places these women within an indeterminate category (28,29). An acute spontaneous abortion is often marked by a beta-hCG level exceeding the DZ without a visible gestational sac by TVUS; in such a case, a falsely positive diagnosis of ectopic pregnancy would be suggested using the DZ criteria (30).

UTERUS

Intrauterine Pregnancy

The sonographic diagnosis of ectopic pregnancy is most commonly made by inclusion, involving direct visualization of an ectopic gestation (27). Alternatively, a diagnosis of exclusion is suggested by the visualization of an IUP (31). Only a remote possibility of a coexistent ectopic pregnancy in the presence of an IUP exists (32). Identification of an IUP on ultrasound in the absence of an adnexal mass is 89% specific for exclusion of an ectopic pregnancy (33).

The TVUS diagnosis of an intrauterine pregnancy (detailed in Table 4.2) can be made as early as $4\frac{1}{2}$ weeks' menstrual age, when a 3-mm gestational sac becomes visible (34–36). The sac is anechoic and spherical, appearing circular in all planes. It is located within the wall of the thickened decidual reaction (37). The high subject contrast between the hyperechoic decidua and the cystic sac augments visibility.

Double Decidual Sign

An intrauterine gestational sac may be confused with a pseudogestational sac (pseudosac) of ectopic pregnancy, a decidual cyst, or a necrotic submucosal leiomyoma (Fig. 4.1) (38,39). The decidua beneath the implantation site of the blastocyst is known as the decidua basalis. The endometrium covering the superficial aspect of the gestational sac is called the decidua capsularis, and the remainder of the endometrium becomes the decidua parietalis. With growth of the pregnancy, the deciduae capsularis and parietalis become directly opposed to one another, separated only by the intervening empty uterine cavity. Ultrasound may reveal this double layer, which forms the double decidual sign (DDS) (38,40).

The DDS appears as dual concentric, hyperechoic, semicircular lines forming a portion of the gestational sac wall (Fig. 4.2). The two decidual

TABLE 4.2

Intrauterine Pregnancy — TVUS Signs

Intradecidual sign (gestational sac within the endometrium, and not within the endometrial cavity)

Double decidual sign

Yolk sac ($5\frac{1}{2}$ weeks)

Embryo

Peritrophoblastic arterial Doppler flow at endomyometrial junction

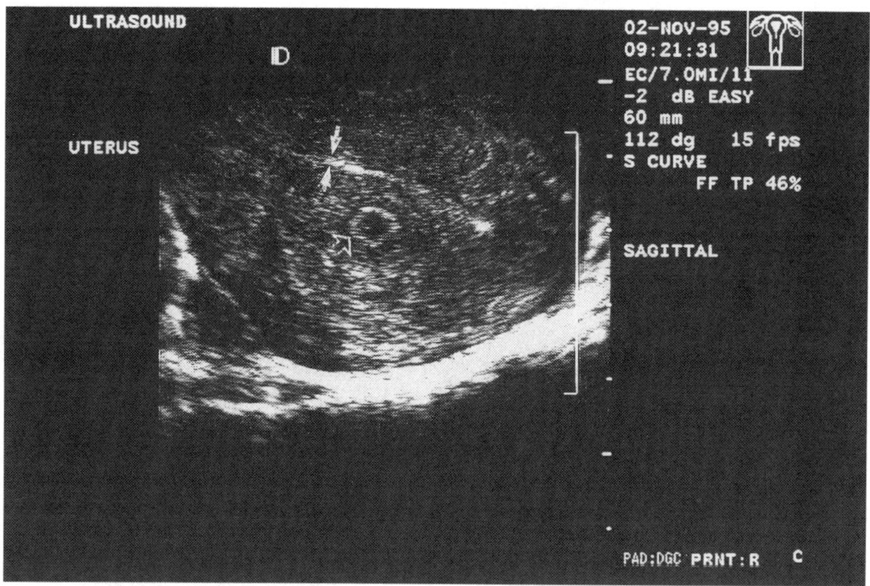

FIG. 4.1.

Gestational sac mimicked by a necrotic uterine leiomyoma. The ring-shaped cystic mass (*open arrow*) is separate from the endometrium (*solid arrows*), verifying a myometrial location.

layers should be of uniform echogenicity and thickness; they should also be discretely marginated. An intervening hypoechoic layer of variable thickness represents the uterine cavity separating the decidual layers. Studies have shown that the DDS appears in 98% of all intrauterine gestational sacs (38). Gestational sacs with a diameter of less than 10 mm may not show the DDS, as their small size results in poor definition of individual decidual layers (41). The degenerating or poorly formed wall of an abnormal IUP (for example, blighted ovum) may lack a DDS (42). A pseudosac with hemorrhage or necrosis centrally within its decidual wall may rarely simulate two decidual layers (38). Nevertheless, despite these pitfalls, the DDS remains the most reliable sign of an IUP prior to visualization of a yolk sac (43).

Uterine Doppler

Chorionic tissue, regardless of its location, appears homogeneously hyperechoic and is indistinguishable from decidualized endometrium on

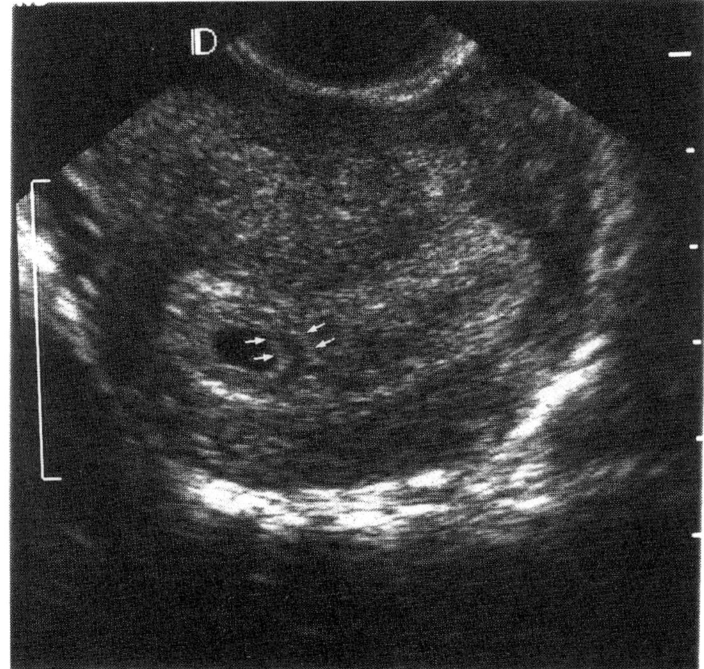

FIG. **4.2.**

A 6-mm intrauterine gestational sac, demonstrating a double decidual sign (*arrows*).

gray-scale images. The supplemental use of Doppler ultrasound provides physiologic evidence of an intrauterine gestational sac by demonstrating peritrophoblastic flow. Significant neovascularity accompanies trophoblastic proliferation, producing high-velocity, low-impedance arterial Doppler flow adjacent to the implantation site. The low impedance results from a large pressure gradient that exists between the maternal spiral arteries and the surrounding low-pressure, smooth-muscle-deficient intervillous spaces of the developing placenta (33,44,45). The vascular changes may be demonstrated with color Doppler as early as 4 1/2 weeks' menstrual age and have a resistive index of less than 0.5, along with spectral broadening indicating turbulent blood flow (32,44,46). Although this type of flow pattern may also appear with submucosal leiomyomas, endometrial cancer, or gestational trophoblastic disease, the differing clinical scenarios should prevent confusion in most cases (9,44,47).

A recent spontaneous abortion may present a confusing TVUS pattern (48,49). A high serum beta-hCG titer without a sonographically apparent gestational sac might suggest the presence of an occult ectopic pregnancy. Color-flow Doppler will demonstrate residual peritrophoblastic flow adjacent to the original implantation site of the gestational sac; this flow can persist for two to three days postabortion (50,51).

Doppler ultrasound creates the in vitro side effects of thermal injury and cavitation, although the same effects have not been well documented in vivo (44,52). The potential harm to the developing pregnancy is theoretical and unquantifiable. A prudent approach is to avoid Doppler interrogation of a normal-appearing intrauterine gestational sac, instead reserving this technique for cases where gray-scale images indicate that the patient is at significant risk for ectopic pregnancy. The benefits accrued by assisting in early diagnosis of ectopic pregnancy supersede the theoretical risks of harmful bioeffects (44).

Endometrium in Ectopic Pregnancy

The endometrial changes associated with an ectopic pregnancy are unpredictable and wide ranging, reflecting the variable hormonal milieu seen in this entity (Fig. 4.3) (53). After examining endometrial histology in 245 cases of ectopic pregnancy, Lopez concluded that any type of endometrium lacking trophoblast could be present. A decidual reaction was found in 42% of these cases, secretory endometrium in 22%, and proliferative endometrium in 12% (54).

Previous ultrasound reports have noted the diversity in endometrial appearance, but found neither thickness nor echogenicity to have predictive value in the diagnosis of ectopic pregnancy (55,56). After intrauterine implantation has produced clinically detectable beta-hCG, the endometrium should follow a late secretory or decidual pattern. The distinctive TVUS appearance of a proliferative or early secretory-phase endometrium occurring in a patient with a positive beta-hCG level should engender a high suspicion of an ectopic pregnancy (see Fig. 4.3B).

Pseudogestational Sac (Pseudosac)

A pseudosac is a collection of simple or complex fluid distending the uterine cavity, outlined by a prominent decidual reaction (see Figs. 4.3F and 4.3G). Such collections are seen in 10% to 20% of ectopic pregnancies, and their presence may be confused with an intrauterine gestational sac (38,44). A pseudosac lies centrally within the uterine cavity, whereas an IUP is eccentric and intradecidual in location (37). A pseudosac conforms to the uterine cavity; it is elliptical or teardrop-shaped, and only rarely spherical. Case reports have noted pseudosacs possessing a simulated DDS, yolk sac, or embryo, although such occurrences remain rare (13,57).

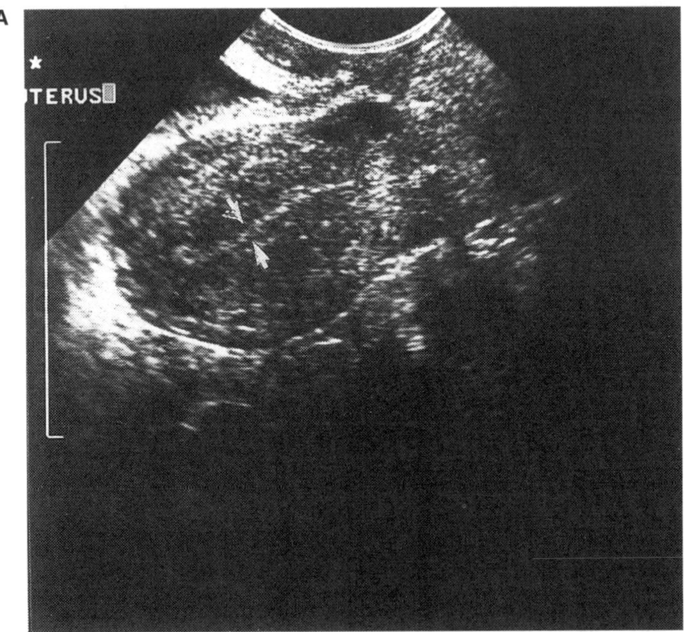

FIG. 4.3.

Endometrial patterns associated with ectopic pregnancy: (A) thin linear, nonstimulated endometrium (*arrows*); (B) three-layered, predominantly hypoechoic late proliferative endometrium (*arrows*); (C) early secretory endometrium (*arrows*) — a decidual cyst (*arrowhead*) is seen superiorly within the endometrium; (D) prominent decidual reaction (*cursors*); (E) complex endometrium echo (*arrows*) — heterogenous material within the uterine cavity represents a combination of sloughed decidua, clot, and free fluid, a pattern that resembles an incomplete abortion; (F) small pseudogestational sac — degenerating decidua surrounding endometrial fluid with a false-positive double decidual sign (*arrows*); (G) large pseudogestational sac (*arrows*) — complex fluid distends the uterine cavity.

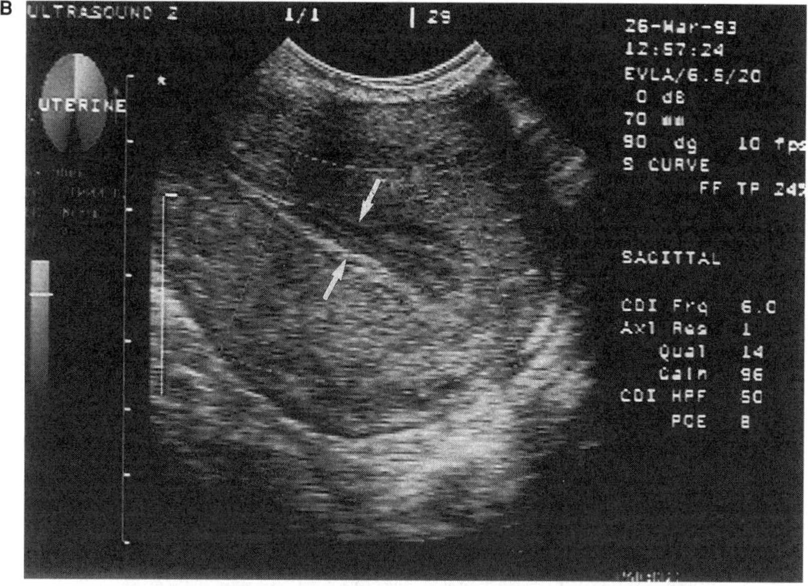

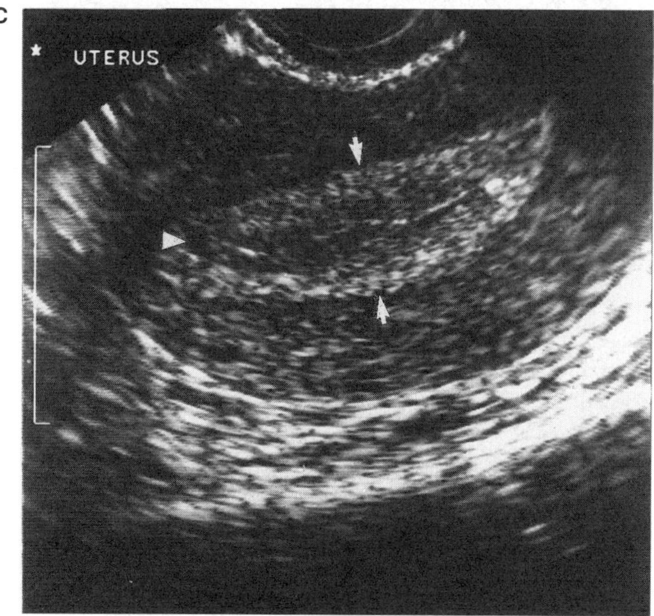

FIG. 4.3.

(*continued*).

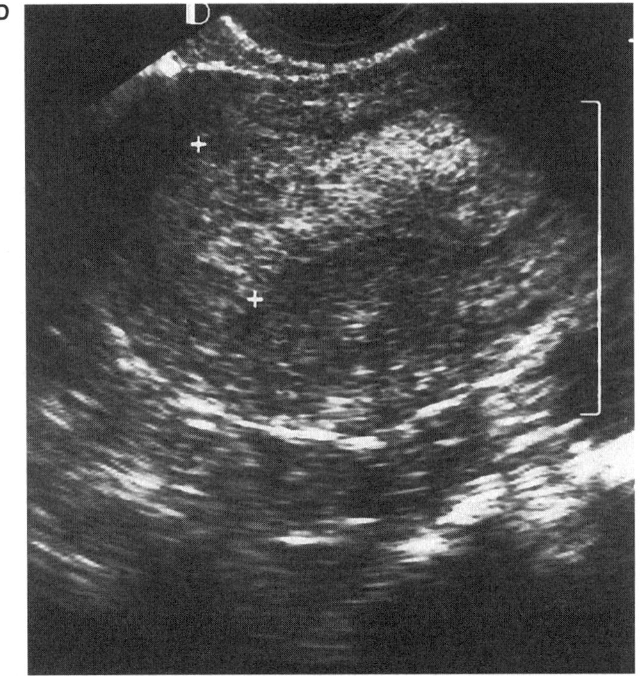

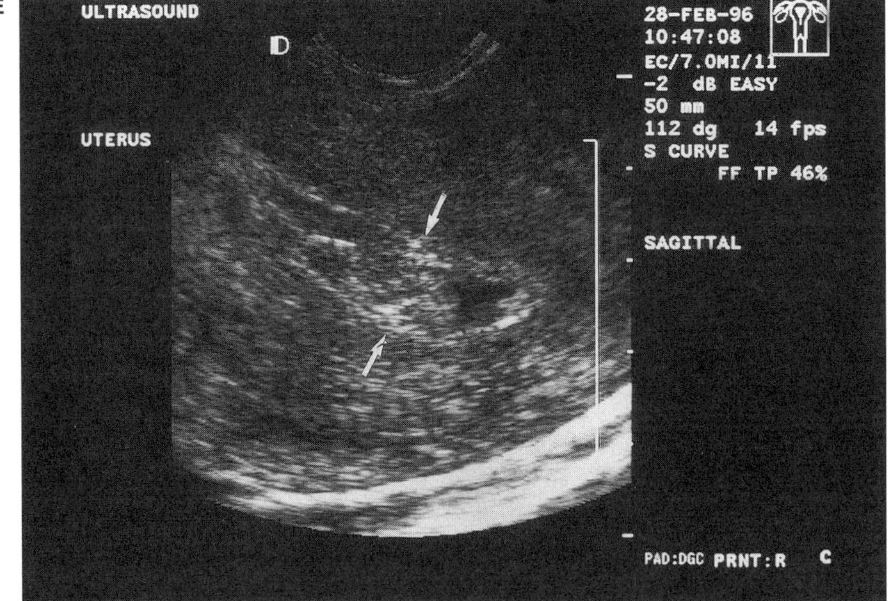

FIG. 4.3.

(*continued*).

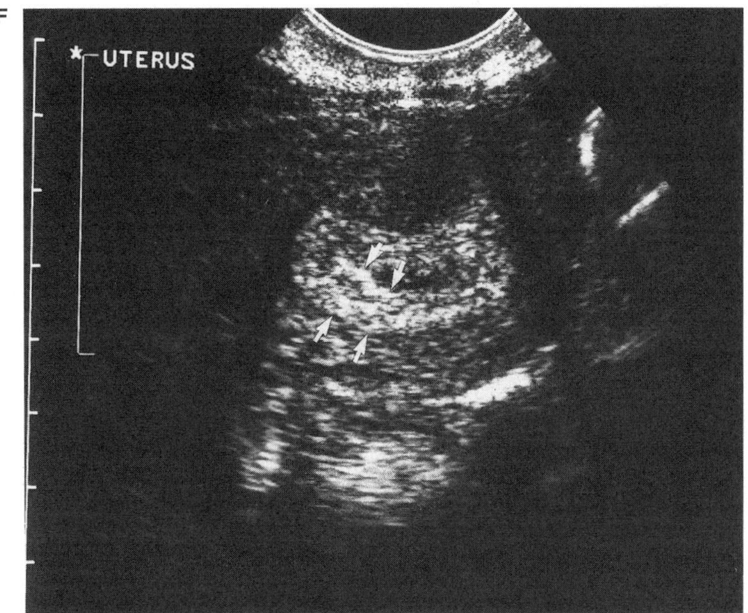

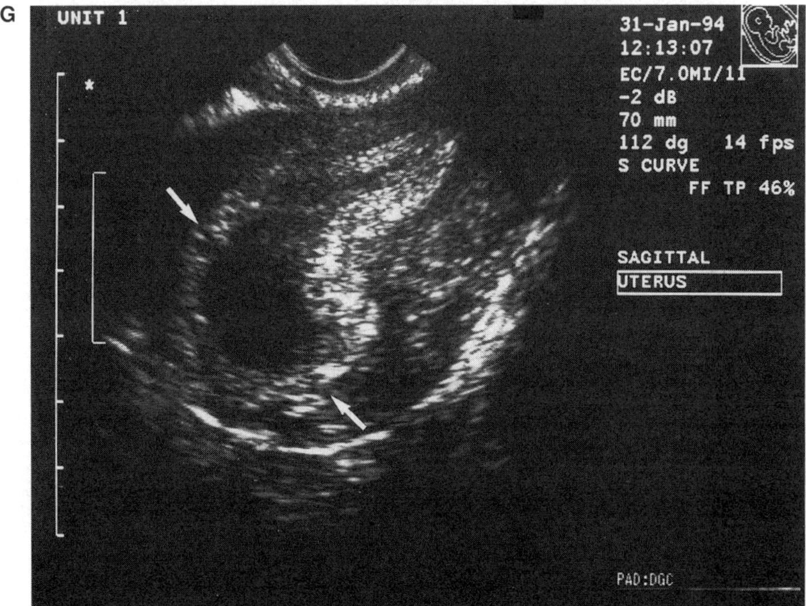

FIG. 4.3.

(continued).

Decidual Cysts

Decidual cysts are small (less than 5 mm in diameter) anechoic cysts typically seen near the endomyometrial junction, and remote from the endometrial canal (see Fig. 4.3C) (39). They are reported in 14% of ectopic pregnancies, but are nonspecific and not diagnostic of ectopic pregnancy.

Doppler Ultrasound of Endometrium in Ectopic Patients

Doppler ultrasound of endometrium in ectopic pregnancy demonstrates absent flow or perhaps minimal venous or high resistance arterial flow (Fig. 4.4) (47). Diagnosis of a pseudosac using pulsed Doppler has achieved a sensitivity of 89% and a specificity of 100% (46). Interrogation of the main uterine artery found no differences in the uterine artery resistance in ectopic pregnancy compared with patients with IUP, although

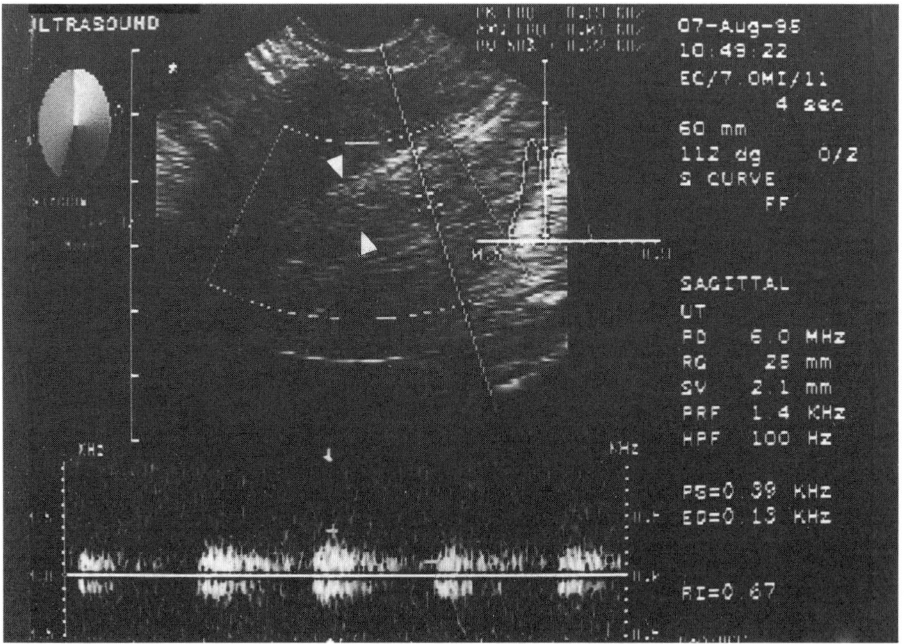

FIG. 4.4.

Uterine blood flow in ectopic pregnancies. Doppler demonstrates sparse periendometrial arterial flow, with nonspecific, high-impedance waveform (*arrowheads* = endometrium).

a diminished uterine artery peak systolic velocity was seen in ectopic pregnancy. This change occurred bilaterally, indicating a systemic rather than local trophoblastic effect, but offered little help in lateralizing the ectopic pregnancy (58).

OVARY

Identification and evaluation of the ovaries are essential in the diagnosis of ectopic pregnancy. The determination of adnexal pathology as intrinsic or extrinsic to the ovary profoundly affects the ultimate diagnosis. In addition, visualization of the ovaries is important because tubal pregnancies appear in close proximity to the ipsilateral ovary.

Corpus Luteum

Virtually all pregnant patients scanned for an ectopic pregnancy will possess a corpus luteum of some activity (Table 4.3). The sonomorphologic and Doppler features of a corpus luteum can appear nearly identical to those following from an ectopic pregnancy (Fig. 4.5) (27). Absence of the corpus luteum is inconsistent with continuation of pregnancy, regardless of its location (9).

Cellular engorgement with lipid deposition is necessary for rapid and profound progesterone synthesis in the corpus luteum (59). These cellular changes are accompanied by intense neoangiogenesis, which originates within the thecal layer that receives considerable ovarian blood flow.

TABLE 4.3

Corpus Luteum — TVUS Patterns

Simple cyst

Cyst with thick wall

Hemorrhagic cyst

Complex or solid appearing hemorrhagic mass

Circumferential flow on color/power Doppler ("ring of fire")

The luteal neovessels are devoid of smooth muscle content, producing a low-resistance arterial circuit (60,61). Color and power Doppler will both demonstrate a characteristic peripheral flow pattern marginating the corpus luteum (Fig. 4.6). The luteal R.I. usually falls in the range of 0.4 to 0.5 (15,62). The Doppler features of a corpus luteum are considerably more uniform than the gray-scale appearance. The diversity of corpus luteal sonographic patterns varies according to the extent of luteal tissue growth, degree of cyst formation, and the presence and age of internal hemorrhage (59). The ovary possessing the corpus luteum is larger than its contralateral pair, with mean respective volumes of 20 cc versus 9 cc (63).

The corpus luteum commonly appears as a simple or complex cyst. This cyst may have either a thin, imperceptible wall or a thick, hyperechoic

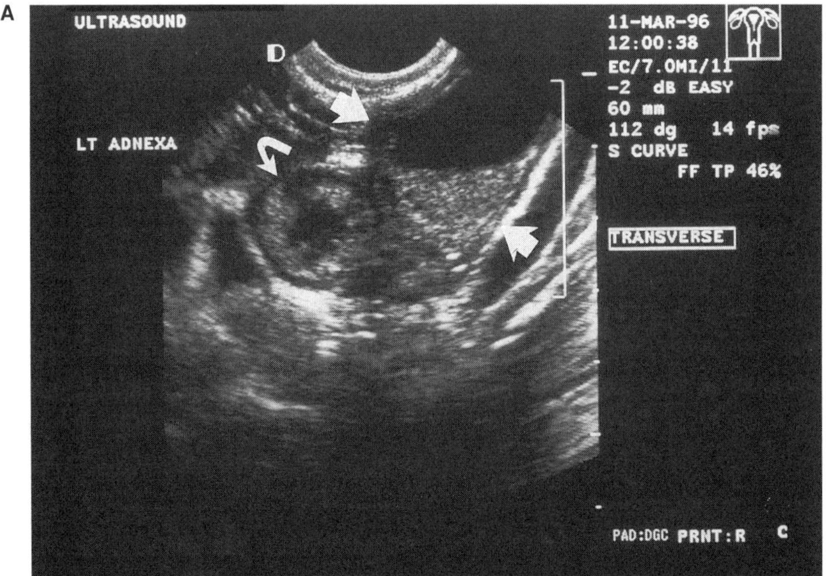

FIG. 4.5.

Ectopic gestational sac versus corpus luteum. (A) The cystic adnexal ring with a thick, hyperechoic wall represents an ectopic pregnancy (*curved arrow*). The sac is adjacent to the ovary (*straight arrows*), which contains a corpus luteum cyst. (B) Exophytic corpus luteum simulating a gestational sac. The ring-shaped adnexal mass (*black arrow*) is definable as corpus luteum only by its continuity with the ovary (*white arrows*).

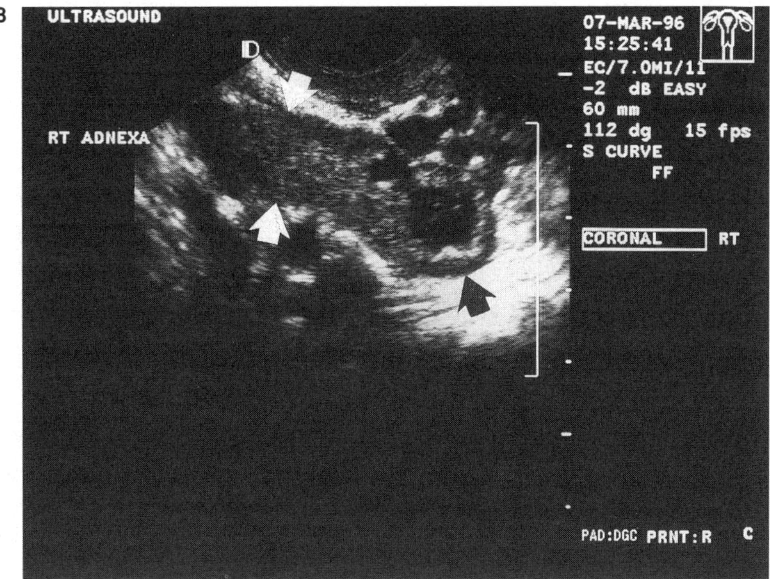

FIG. 4.5.

(*continued*).

or hypoechoic wall, with irregular areas of internal amorphous solid material and septations within the cyst representing hemorrhage (see Fig. 4.5B). In addition, a corpus luteum may assume the appearance of a solid mass, being hypoechoic, isoechoic, or hyperechoic to the ovarian parenchyma (59). An isoechoic corpus luteum may not be apparent on the gray-scale images, becoming conspicuous only on color Doppler.

Multiple studies have failed to find any direct correlation between luteal impedance and gestational age of the pregnancy (58). No differences in luteal impedance have been noted between IUP and ectopic pregnancies either, despite the uniformly lower progesterone levels seen in ectopic pregnancy (58,62). These studies infer that the luteal circulatory changes apparent through Doppler ultrasound are not directly related to hormonal function. A higher luteal R.I. (0.58) was noted in involuting ectopic pregnancies compared with the R.I. (0.39) in developing ectopic pregnancies (7).

A corpus luteum contralateral to the ectopic pregnancy occurs in 11% to 20% of cases. The frequency of this occurrence limits its use as a marker for the side of an ectopic pregnancy (63–65).

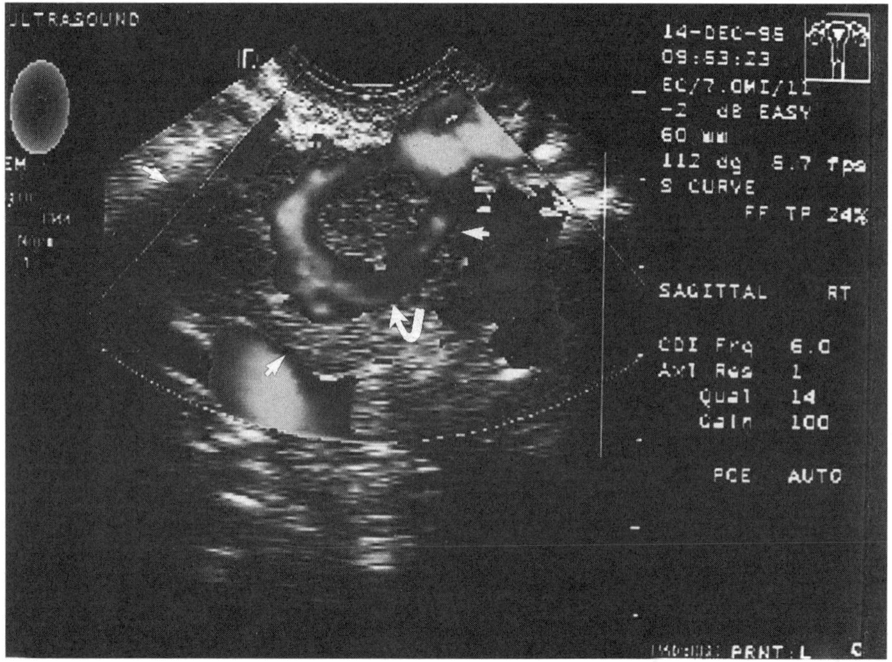

FIG. 4.6.

Corpus luteum, power Doppler. The circular area of vascular flow, the "ring of fire" (*curved arrow*), delineates a hypoechoic intraovarian mass (*small arrows* = ovary).

Multiple corpora lutea secondary to multiple ovulation may occur, especially in assisted reproduction patients; this development may indicate that the patient has an increased risk for heterotopic pregnancy (Fig. 4.7) (59).

Nonphysiologic Ovarian Masses

Nonphysiologic ovarian masses are uncommonly found in pregnant patients, with masses requiring surgical intervention reported in 1 of 1300 live births (Fig. 4.8) (66). An ipsilateral ovarian mass may obscure or be confused with a coexistent ectopic pregnancy, preventing TVUS diagnosis. Distinguishing features include the intraovarian location, nongestational sac-like appearance, and better-defined margins of a complex ovarian mass compared with an ectopic pregnancy.

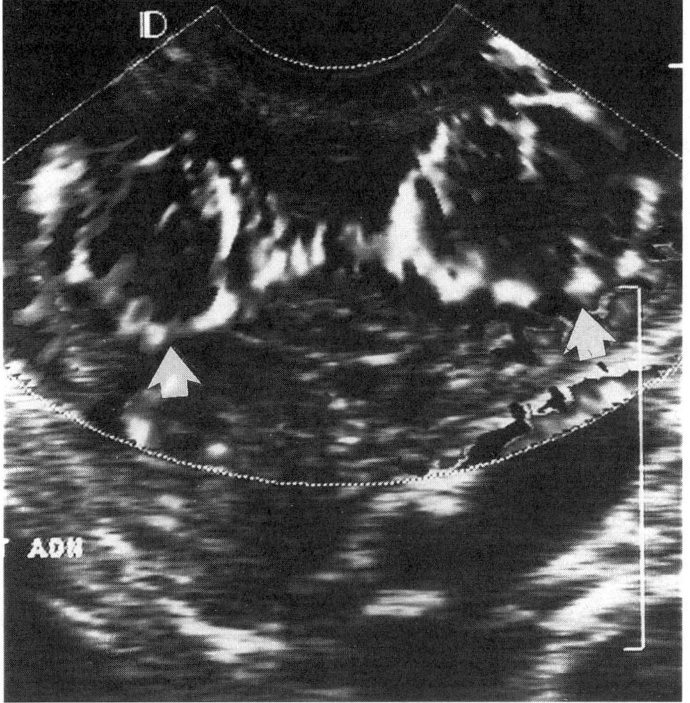

FIG. 4.7.

Dual ipsilateral corpora lutea. The power Doppler topogram demonstrates two ring-like vascular ovarian masses (*arrows*).

ADNEXA

The key criterion in the TVUS diagnosis of ectopic pregnancy is the identification of any extraovarian mass that is not a simple cyst (67). The spectrum of TVUS appearances of ectopic pregnancy will be described in order of descending specificity (Table 4.4).

Live Ectopic Pregnancy

Sonographic visualization of cardiac activity within an extrauterine embryo is 100% specific for an ectopic pregnancy (63). The relative proportion of live ectopics seen with TVUS has declined in recent years, as improved

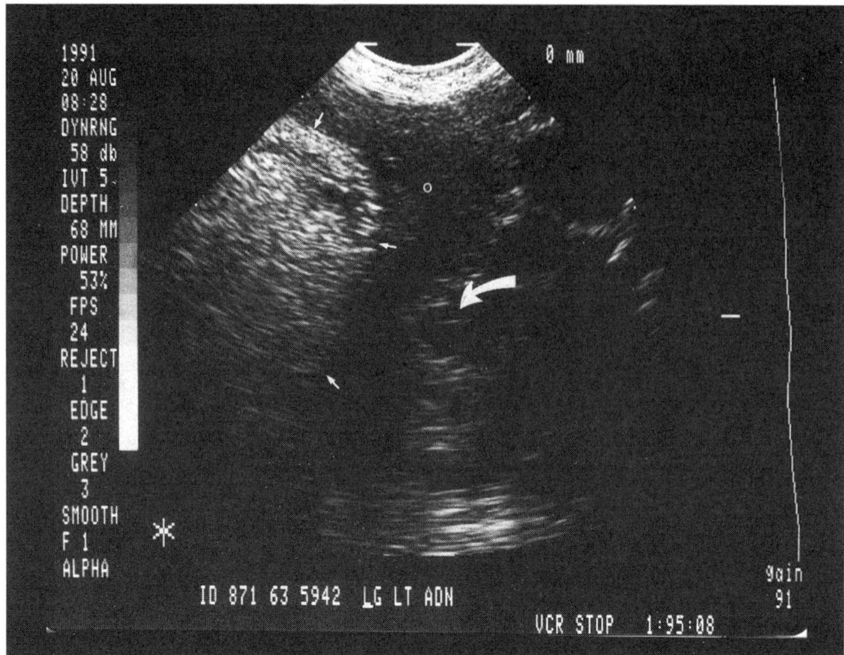

FIG. 4.8.

Coexistent ectopic pregnancy and ovarian neoplasm. The large hyperechoic mass (*small arrows*) represents a teratoma originating from the ovary (*o*). An ectopic gestational sac (*curved arrow*) is seen posterior to the ovary.

sensitivity has enabled diagnosis of more subtle lesions (56). Cardiac activity is readily detectable with the naked eye, using real-time ultrasound, videotape, m-mode, or Doppler to document the findings (10). Frame-to-frame averaging, a processing feature available on most ultrasound machines, can obscure cardiac motion by excessive smoothing of the image. This feature should be lowered or disabled in very small embryos or embryos with slow heart rates. The presence of cardiac activity also affects the treatment choice, as patients harboring a live ectopic pregnancy have a significantly higher rate of nonsurgical treatment failure (68–72).

Ectopic Gestational Sac

An ectopic gestational sac has a hyperechoic, thick (2- to 5-mm) wall with a central sonolucent lumen (see Fig. 4.5A) (70,73). An embryo or yolk sac may be present internally but is more often absent, as the deficient

TABLE 4.4

Ectopic Pregnancy — TVUS Appearances

Ectopic gestational sac (adnexal ring)
Empty sac
± Yolk sac or embryo
± Cardiac activity

Complex extraovarian mass
Hematosalpinx

Hemoperitoneum
Simple
Echogenic fluid
Indefinite uterus

Normal TVUS exam
If ovaries are not identified on the TVUS exam, a TAS evaluation is required

Peritrophoblastic flow on Doppler
Vascularity ranges from none to extreme hypervascularity
Impedance ranges from low to intermediate-high resistance

vascular supply of the ectopic sac results in abnormal development (17). The ectopic gestational sac, which is also known as an adnexal ring, has a high specificity for ectopic pregnancy (74). TVUS can visualize an ectopic gestational sac as small as 5 mm in diameter (Fig. 4.9) (75).

Complex Adnexal Mass

An ectopic pregnancy can also appear as a heterogeneous mass, composed of interspersed hypoechoic and hyperechoic tissue (Fig. 4.10). The complex mass consists of blood and trophoblast, with the appearance varying with the relative proportion of each component (76,77). A wide range of beta-hCG levels may be seen with an adnexal mass of a given size because of the variable amount of blood clot present (Fig. 4.11) (73).

Despite the featureless, nonspecific architecture of a complex mass, diagnostic accuracy is achieved by demonstrating its extraovarian location,

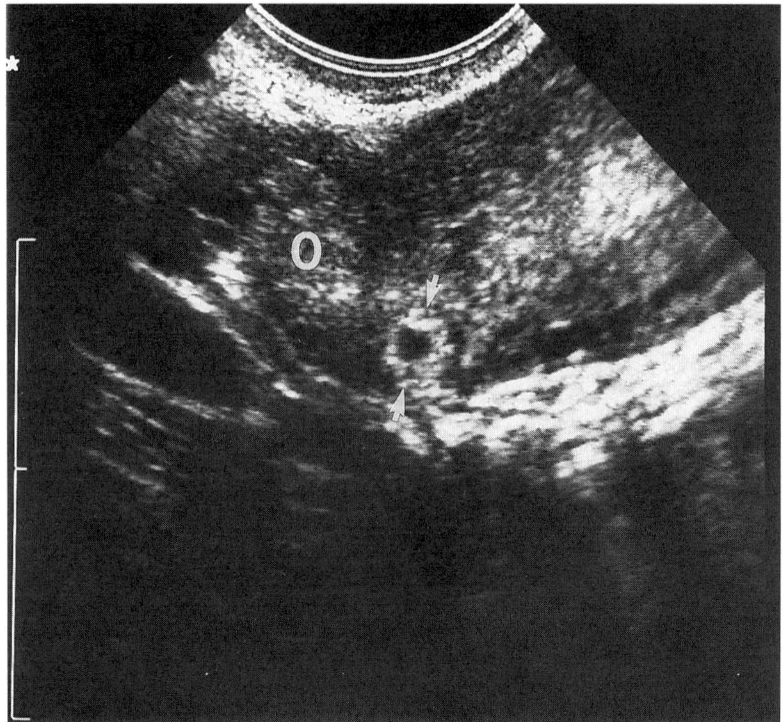

FIG. 4.9.

Small ectopic pregnancy. The 7-mm extrauterine gestational sac (*arrows*) lies medial to ovary (*o*) and lateral to the uterus.

as similar-appearing complex masses may appear within the ovary, such as hemorrhagic cysts or neoplasms (33). A thin-walled simple cyst, regardless of its location or clinical presentation, is unlikely to represent an ectopic pregnancy (67).

Larger complex masses with extensive hemorrhage may prevent identification of the ovary. Nevertheless, the presence of a mass, free peritoneal fluid, and clinical suspicion of an ectopic pregnancy should enable the correct diagnosis.

Hematosalpinx

A hematosalpinx — a subset of a complex mass — has a tubular or round shape representing the accumulation of blood and trophoblast within a distended intact fallopian tube (Fig. 4.12) (56). A hematosalpinx may

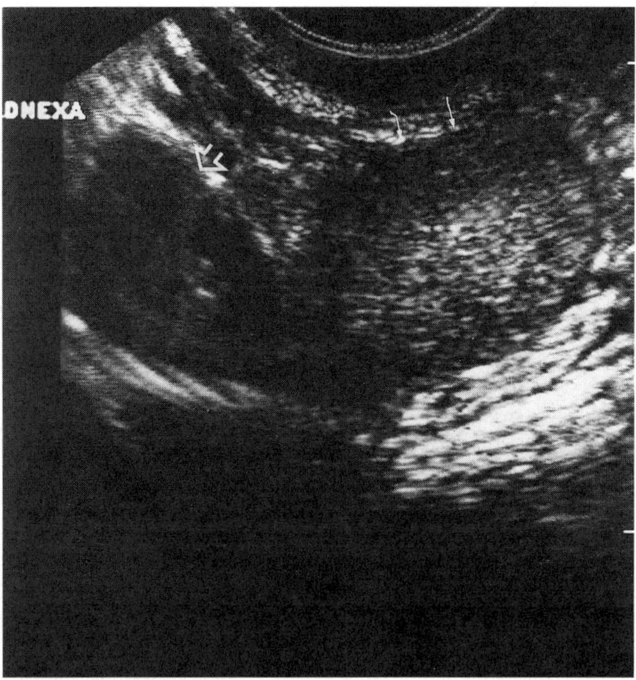

FIG. 4.10.

Ectopic pregnancy appearing as a complex mass. The solid-appearing round mass (*arrows*) is separate from the ovary (*open arrow*).

be isoechoic to the ovary, appearing on TVUS as asymmetric ovarian enlargement (78). This sign is not very accurate, as the ovaries will commonly be asymmetric because the presence of the corpus luteum (63). An array of follicles delineates the cortical surface of a normal ovary. A tubal mass will be located superficial to the follicles, confirming an extraovarian location.

Cul-de-Sac Fluid

TVUS's high sensitivity for the detection of cul-de-sac fluid has essentially rendered culdocentesis an obsolete procedure (75,79–81). The TVUS exam is performed in the supine position with an empty bladder, allowing fluid to collect unimpeded within the cul-de-sac, which is the most dependent portion of the peritoneal cavity (82). Peritoneal fluid may be characterized as simple or echogenic. Echogenic fluid has been attributed to hemoperitoneum, whereas simple anechoic fluid is nonspecific in nature (83).

The visualization of diffuse internal echoes within fluid is highly dependent on using the proper sonographic technique (Fig. 4.13). Low-power or low-gain settings will obscure echoes, whereas high-gain settings will create artifactual echoes. Particle motion seen with real-time ultrasound is considered specific for echogenic fluid; this motion may be spontaneous from active bleeding or elicited by movement or manual compression of the patient's anterior abdominal wall (83).

Cul-de-sac fluid has been observed in 21% to 95% of ectopic pregnancies diagnosed with TVUS (16,34,83,84). Fluid also appears in more than 20% of normal IUPs, attributable to intrauterine hemorrhage

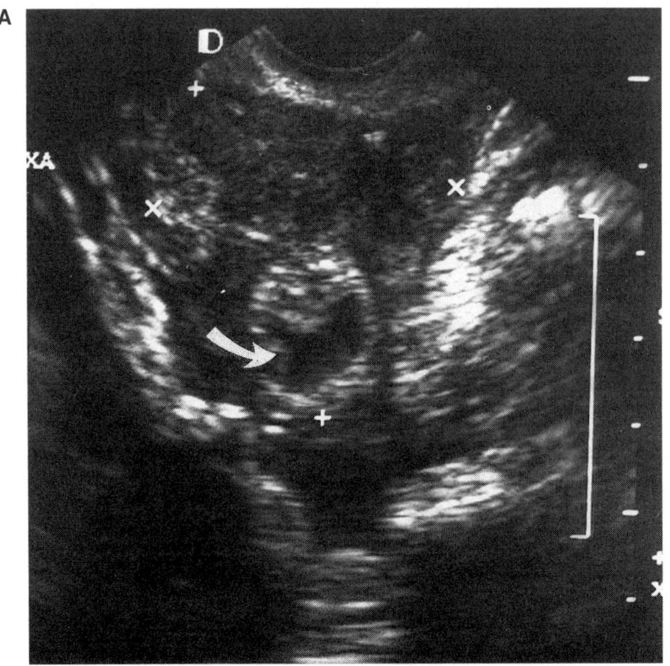

FIG. 4.11.

Complex ectopic pregnancy. (A) This large adnexal mass (*cursors*) is predominantly hypoechoic, representing hemorrhage. A central hyperechoic component (*curved arrow*) represents a gestational sac remnant. (B) Power Doppler shows the avascularity of the hemorrhagic region (*solid arrows*). Peripheral flow (R.I. = 0.62) surrounds the area of residual trophoblast (*open arrow*).

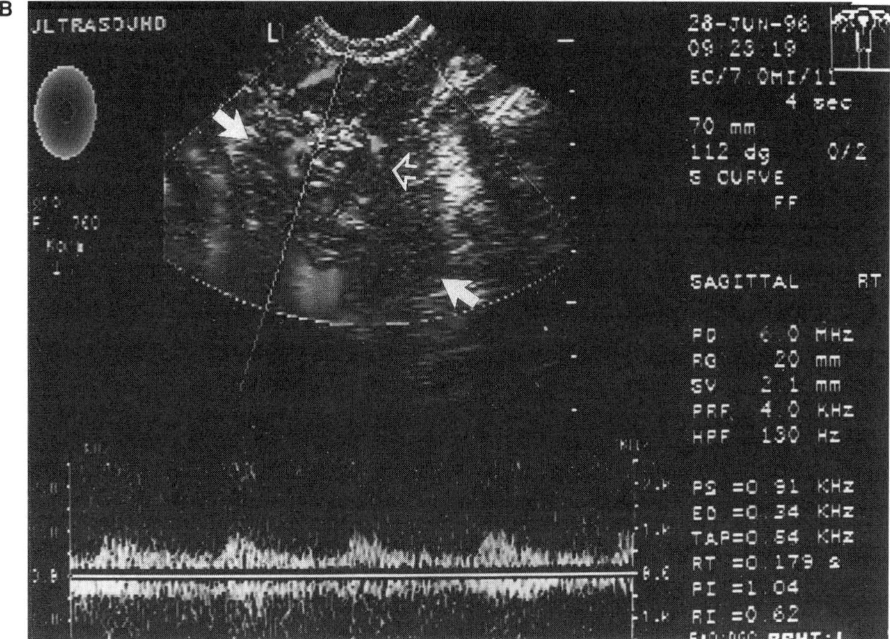

FIG. 4.11.

(*continued*).

with retrograde flow through the fallopian tubes or from a ruptured corpus luteum cyst (16,85).

Severe intraperitoneal hemorrhage will extend into the paracolic gutter and subhepatic space, both of which are located beyond the range of the TVUS probe. Acute clotted blood is similar in echogenicity to the myometrium, and large amounts of acute hemorrhage may mask the uterine contour. This process creates an "indefinite uterus sign," where the uterus may be identified only by locating the endometrial echo (Fig. 4.14) (86).

Pelvic hemorrhage ascends the right paracolic gutter preferentially over the shallower left gutter. The phrenico-colic ligament serves as a barrier to drainage of left paracolic gutter fluid into the upper-left quadrant; the right gutter, on the other hand, drains freely into Morrison's pouch. Expansion of the rib cage during inspiration produces negative pressure in the upper abdomen, creating a pressure gradient between the upper and lower peritoneal cavity. This pressure gradient, which

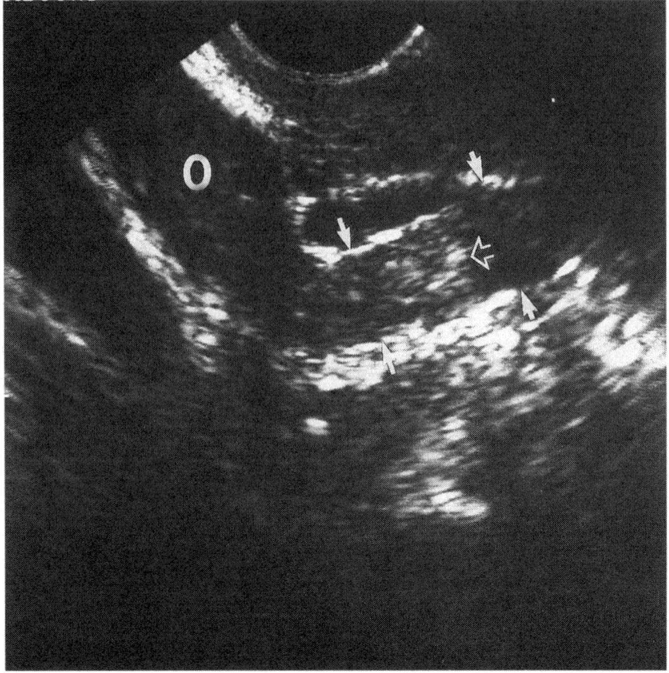

FIG. 4.12.

Hematosalpinx. This oblong adnexal mass (*solid arrows*) results from a fallopian tube distended with hemorrhage. A central hyperechoic focus (*open arrow*) within the mass is an area of residual trophoblast (*o* = ovary).

is accentuated when the patient is in an upright position, provides a hydrostatic mechanism for extension of pelvic fluid into the abdomen, irrespective of the patient's position (87). The negative upper abdominal pressure also induces a sedimentation effect on pelvic hemorrhagic fluid that is being drawn into the abdomen. The fluid that accumulates in the upper abdomen has a lower hematocrit and appears anechoic on ultrasound. The high subject contrast between the liver and anechoic blood creates greater visibility of the abdominal fluid compared with the echogenic clotted pelvic hemorrhage (Fig. 4.15).

Normal TVUS

A normal TVUS in the setting of an ectopic pregnancy occurs with an estimated incidence of 3% to 19% (30,67,74,81,85). Patients with falling

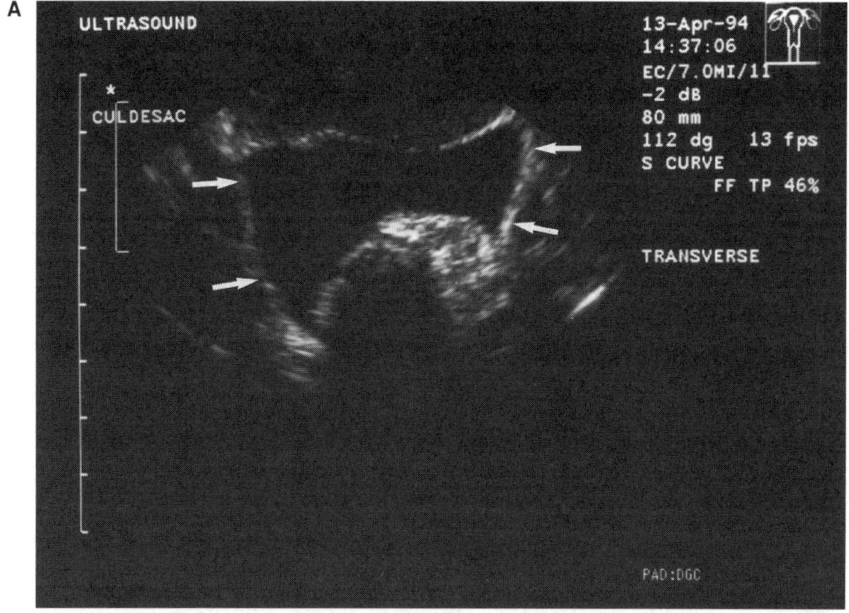

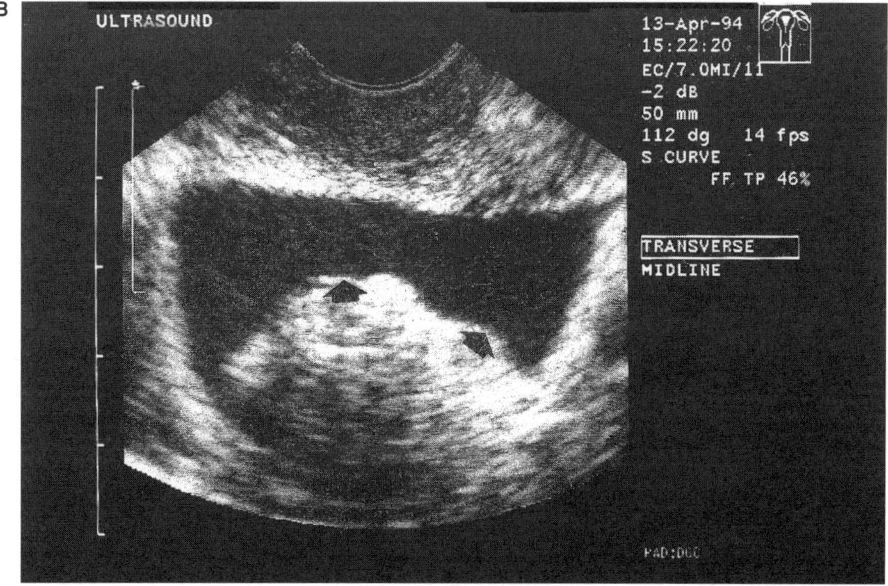

FIG. 4.13.

Hemoperitoneum. (A) Simple-appearing cul-de-sac fluid (*arrows*). (B) Same patient as part A. Optimized gain settings reveal diffuse, internal particulate echoes (*arrows*).

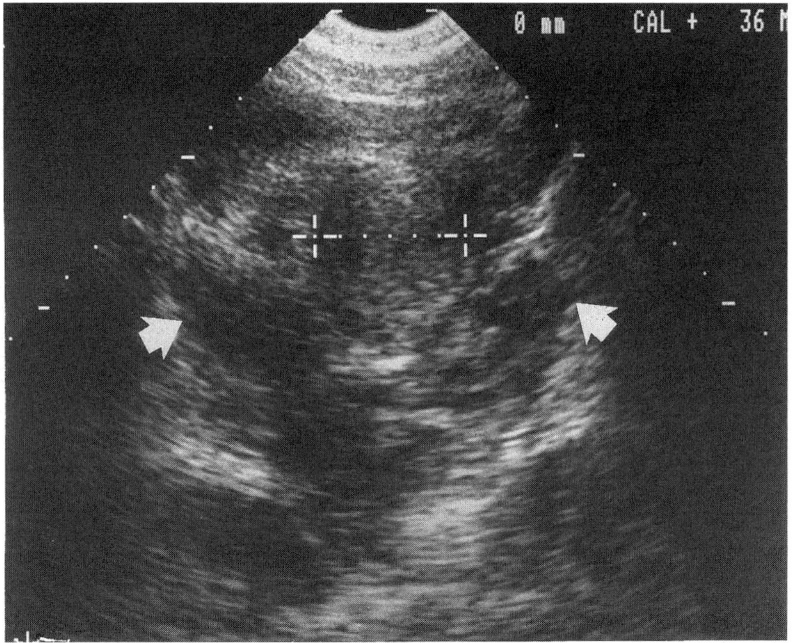

FIG. 4.14.

Severe hemoperitoneum. A TAS scan shows the uterus (*cursors*) engulfed and camouflaged by a large, hemorrhagic pelvic mass (*arrows*), producing the indefinite uterus sign.

serum beta-hCG levels and normal TVUS examinations may be followed expectantly and classified as having trophoblast in regression (88).

Hahlin observed 80 patients with abnormal serial beta-hCG titers and with nonvisualization of an IUP or ectopic pregnancy using TVUS (89). Of these cases, 56% were classified as trophoblast in regression, and 20% required surgery for an ectopic pregnancy. Those patients with falling beta-hCG levels and low progesterone levels had a 97% spontaneous regression rate.

Adnexal Doppler

Doppler evaluation of ectopic pregnancy has been hampered by inter-observer and technical variabilities, both of which affect reproducibility of results. In particular, a substantial learning curve exists for accurate Doppler application (48).

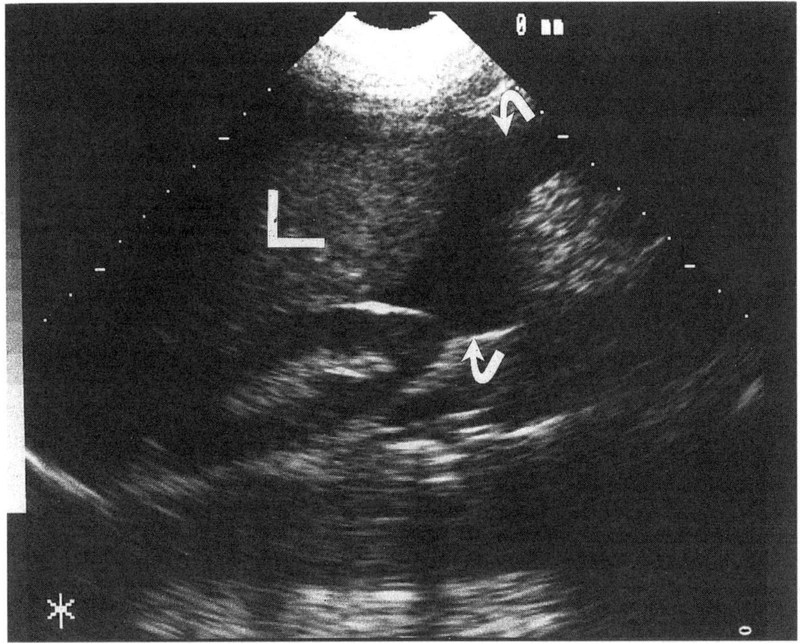

FIG. **4.15.**

Severe hemoperitoneum. Same patient as Figure 4.14. Note the large amount of anechoic fluid within Morison's pouch (*curved arrows*) (L = liver).

As with an IUP, peritrophoblastic flow may be seen in association with ectopic pregnancy, producing high–amplitude, low–impedance arterial flow and variable venous flow (Fig. 4.16) (18,71). Significantly greater variation is seen in the amount and impedance of ectopic peritrophoblastic flow compared with intrauterine peritrophoblastic flow, reflecting the erratic growth and viability of ectopic tissue (31,90). A fall in resistance has been noted with progressive trophoblastic growth. An R.I. ranging between 0.6 and 0.36 has been demonstrated in ectopic tissue (31,64,77). The variable impedances noted with ectopic pregnancy hamper use of the R.I. in distinguishing ectopic pregnancies from other adnexal masses (see Fig. 4.11B).

A loose correlation is seen between beta-hCG titers and the vascularity of an ectopic pregnancy, as both are directly related to the volume of active trophoblast. Tekay found that more than 88% of ectopic pregnancies demonstrating positive flow on color Doppler had a quantitative beta-hCG level exceeding 800 mIU/mL (IRP) (77). Ectopic pregnancies that demonstrate Doppler flow tend to be larger and more closely simulate normal development; in one study, color Doppler flow was seen in 71% of adnexal rings but in only 29% of complex masses (77). The color Doppler flow pattern is most striking in those ectopic pregnancies with obvious gray-scale findings. Ectopic pregnancies with low beta-hCG levels and minimal real-time findings are unlikely to demonstrate prominent Doppler flow. In one study involving only ectopic pregnancies with falling beta-hCG titers, only 50% of this population showed positive Doppler flow (91). Doppler identification of an ectopic pregnancy that is not visible on gray-scale ultrasound is a rare event, reported as being 1 in 65 cases (92).

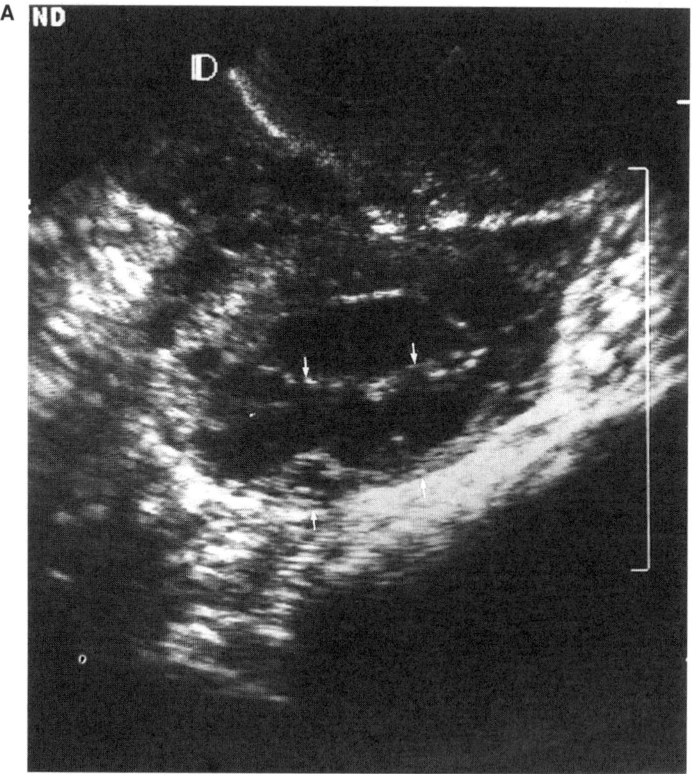

FIG. 4.16.

Hypervascular ectopic pregnancy. (A) An adnexal ring (*arrows*) with a thick hyperechoic wall. (B) Power Doppler shows large venous structures comprising the gestational sac wall.

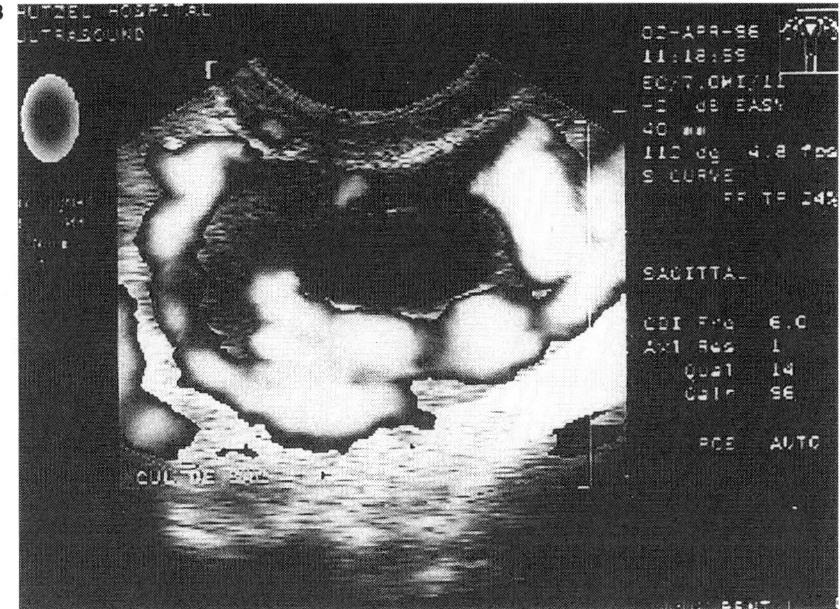

FIG. 4.16.

(*continued*).

A difference was noted in impedances of histologically determined developing ectopic pregnancies compared with those of involuting ectopic pregnancies. Lower R.I.s were seen in the developing group (mean = 0.39) compared with the involuting group (mean = 0.51) (7).

Studies showing a significant improvement in the diagnostic accuracy for ectopic pregnancy by adding color Doppler to TVUS were compromised by overly restrictive criteria for the gray-scale diagnosis (47,64). Achiron demonstrated only 48% sensitivity for ectopic pregnancy using color Doppler; the imaging technique provided no more information than the use of gray-scale images alone in stable patients (33).

TVUS Accuracy in Diagnosis of Ectopic Pregnancy

Brown analyzed positivity criteria from 10 studies that used TVUS to diagnose ectopic pregnancy (67). The single most accurate sign was an extraovarian adnexal mass. A complex mass was a considerably more sensitive (84%) diagnostic sign than a live embryo (20%) or a gestational sac (65%). The high sensitivity of a complex mass resulted in little sacrifice of specificity (99% versus 100% for both a live ectopic pregnancy and a gestational sac).

False-Positive Diagnosis of Ectopic Pregnancy

Table 4.5 details etiologies of false-positive TVUS for ectopic pregnancy. A necrotic subserosal uterine leiomyoma, bowel, pelvic infection, ovarian neoplasm, or corpus luteum may all simulate ectopic pregnancy on TVUS (Figs. 4.5B and 4.17) (35,56,93). A bowel loop in cross section appears ring-like, but peristalsis and elongation on an orthogonal view should prevent confusion with ectopic pregnancy. A ruptured corpus luteum cyst creates an adnexal clot and peritoneal fluid indistinguishable from a complex ectopic adnexal mass (Fig. 4.18) (35).

Acute pelvic inflammatory disease can create a complex tubal mass with echogenic, purulent cul-de-sac fluid and low-resistance Doppler flow. The diagnosis can usually be achieved clinically.

TVUS is very successful at distinguishing ovarian masses from extra-ovarian masses. Ballottement of the mass performed between the TVUS probe and the examiner's hand placed on the anterior abdomen will show an intraovarian mass moving in unison with the ovary. An extraovarian mass will slide on the ovary with manual pressure.

TABLE 4.5

Etiologies of False-Positive TVUS for Ectopic Pregnancy

Corpus luteum
   Exophytic
   Thick-walled cyst
   Ruptured
Ovarian neoplasm
Pelvic inflammatory disease
Endometriosis
Bowel
Pedunculated necrotic uterine leiomyoma

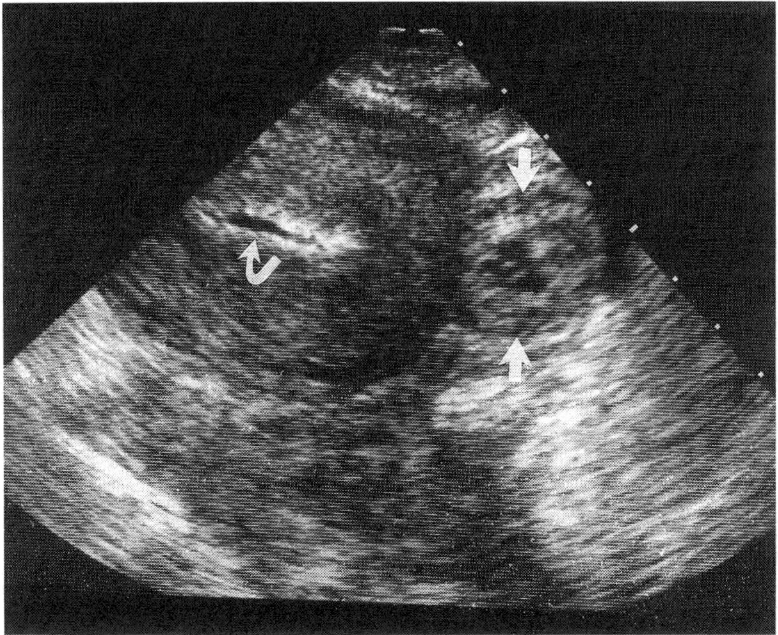

FIG. 4.17.

False-positive TVUS diagnosis of ectopic pregnancy. An apparent ectopic gestational sac (*arrows*) containing a yolk sac is located adjacent to the lateral uterine wall. A pedunculated uterine leiomyoma was found at laparoscopy (*curved arrow* = endometrium).

False-Negative Diagnosis of Ectopic Pregnancy

Table 4.6 details etiologies of false-negative TVUS for ectopic pregnancy. Very small tubal pregnancies or those located high in the pelvis may be missed on TVUS (74). An ectopic pregnancy may be obscured or displaced by a coexistent pelvic mass (9). Extensive pelvic adhesions may prevent adequate adnexal visualization.

Large leiomyomatous uteri pose an especially difficult challenge. Distortion and displacement of the endometrium may prevent visualization of an early IUP, and evaluation of the adnexae is limited because of displacement of the fallopian tubes and ovaries. A careful TAS is essential in these patients, along with close clinical monitoring.

Fallopian Tube Rupture

Earlier TVUS reports, involving limited numbers of patients, attained a successful diagnosis of tubal rupture based on the presence of more than

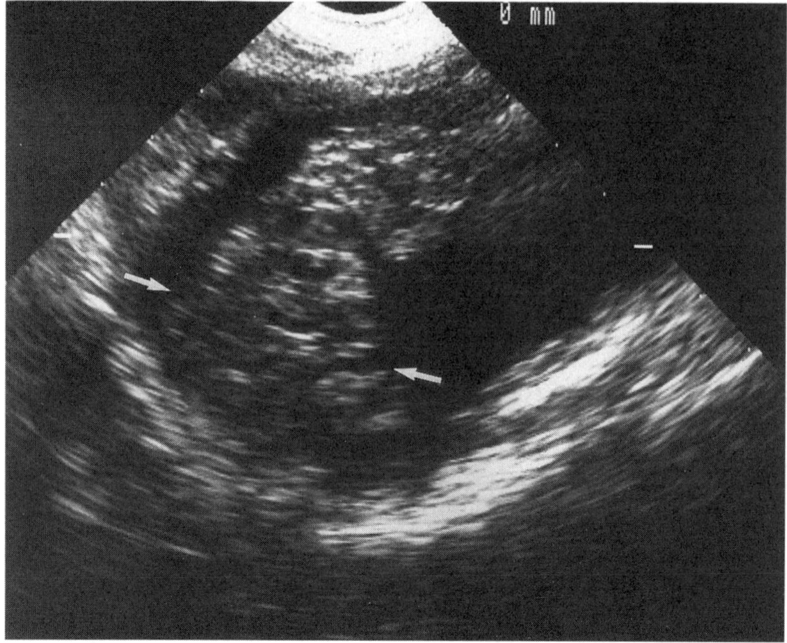

FIG. 4.18.

Ruptured corpus luteum cyst. A complex adnexal mass (*arrows*) is surrounded by peritoneal fluid — findings highly suggestive of an ectopic pregnancy. At surgery a blood clot from a ruptured luteal cyst was found.

TABLE 4.6

Etiologies of False-Negative TVUS for Ectopic Pregnancy

Small size of ectopic pregnancy

Leiomyomatous uterus

High pelvic position of the ectopic pregnancy

Large ovarian mass

Extensive pelvic adhesions

Ectopic pregnancy mistaken for corpus luteum

Bowel gas (ileus)

Uncooperative patient

minimal cul-de-sac fluid, a large adnexal mass, or absence of an intact gestational sac (75). Multiple studies describe the nonspecificity of even large amounts of peritoneal fluid for tubal rupture (35,56).

Frates described a series of 132 patients diagnosed with an ectopic pregnancy by TVUS with supplemental TAS to quantify intraperitoneal fluid (94). Each patient underwent laparoscopic assessment of tubal integrity. No differences were found in the tubal rupture rate in patients with an intact ectopic gestational sac versus those with a complex adnexal mass. The mean size of adnexal masses was larger in the ruptured group, albeit with considerable overlap. The smallest mass seen with tubal rupture measured 1 cm in size, and nearly one-third of masses smaller than 3.5 cm were associated with tubal rupture. In 37% of cases with severe hemoperitoneum on ultrasound (fluid extending into abdomen), patients were found to have intact fallopian tubes at surgery. In addition, 21% of patients with minimal or no cul-de-sac fluid had ruptured fallopian tubes. No differences in the echogenicity of fluid were observed between the ruptured and unruptured women. All sonographically identified fluid — whether echogenic or simple — was found to represent hemoperitoneum at surgery. Active hemorrhage was surgically visualized as emanating from the fimbriated end of the fallopian tube in patients with hemoperitoneum and intact tubes.

In Sadek's series of 57 ectopic pregnancies seen on TVUS, 96% of patients had hemoperitoneum and 91% of patients had intact fallopian tubes (84). Given that clinical data show a positive culdocentesis in 77% of ectopic pregnancies with intact fallopian tubes, these results suggest caution in attempts to sonographically assess tubal integrity (79).

Conservative Therapy and Ultrasound

Medical and conservative surgical therapy have largely replaced salpingectomy in patients with unruptured ectopic pregnancies desirous of future fertility (3). Earlier diagnosis of ectopic pregnancy with beta-hCG values and TVUS has resulted in an increased percentage of unruptured tubal pregnancies at presentation (82,84,95).

Although inclusion criteria for nonsurgical therapies have not been standardized, most rely on beta-hCG titers and TVUS parameters such as adnexal mass size, no evidence of tubal rupture, and absent cardiac activity (96–100). Whereas low and falling beta-hCG levels usually constitute evidence for ectopic pregnancy involution, tubal rupture requiring emergency surgery in the presence of low levels of beta-hCG has been reported (101).

Serial TVUS exams have been performed on nonsurgically treated ectopic pregnancy patients. They demonstrate the highly variable patterns of a resolving ectopic pregnancy. A residual adnexal mass is typically identified, persisting as long as eight weeks after the patient receives a local methotrexate injection (71,72,98). Initial post-therapeutic enlargement of the ectopic mass is usually seen, peaking at one day after initiation of therapy (72,101–103). Treatment failure is predicted by persistent and progressive enlargement of the adnexal mass, whereas diminished mass size at one week postdiagnosis is predictive of an adequate response (91).

Results from attempts to use Doppler to monitor conservative therapy have proved disappointing. Atri found that 68% of ectopic pregnancies became more vascular after methotrexate therapy, and 44% of spontaneously regressing ectopic pregnancies subsequently developed Doppler vascularity, despite the absence of initial flow (72,102). Cacciatore found no appreciable differences in initial or post-treatment Doppler flow when assessing patients responding to and those refractory to medical therapy (91). A progressive rise in resistance was noted in resolving ectopic pregnancies, with R.I. values increasing from a mean of 0.26 to a mean of 0.81 at 45 days postinjection. The diverse and nonspecific morphologic and vascular changes seen in conservatively treated patients, therefore, limit the value of TVUS in monitoring response to therapy.

Persistent Ectopic Pregnancy

Continued growth and enlargement of residual tubal trophoblastic tissue following conservative ectopic pregnancy therapy constitutes a persistent ectopic pregnancy (79,104). The incidence varies from 1.4% to 20%, reflecting the absence of uniform protocols for serum beta-hCG titer monitoring of conservatively treated patients (3,65,103). Approximately one-half of reported cases are diagnosed by abnormal beta-hCG titers, with the remaining patients presenting with acute symptomatology (3). Patients who are not closely monitored or lost to follow-up have a greater risk of tubal rupture and hemoperitoneum-induced hypovolemia (102,103).

TVUS can demonstrate recurrent trophoblastic tissue that appears as an irregular, complex, hyperechoic mass (Fig. 4.19). Hypervascular peritrophoblastic flow appears at the periphery of the mass. The recurrent trophoblast is usually located at the original anatomic site, but may sometimes be dispersed throughout the peritoneal cavity (103).

HETEROTOPIC PREGNANCIES

The identification of an IUP greatly reduces but does not eliminate the possibility of an ectopic pregnancy. Recorded rates of heterotopic pregnancies have risen from 1 per 30,000 pregnancies in 1948 to more

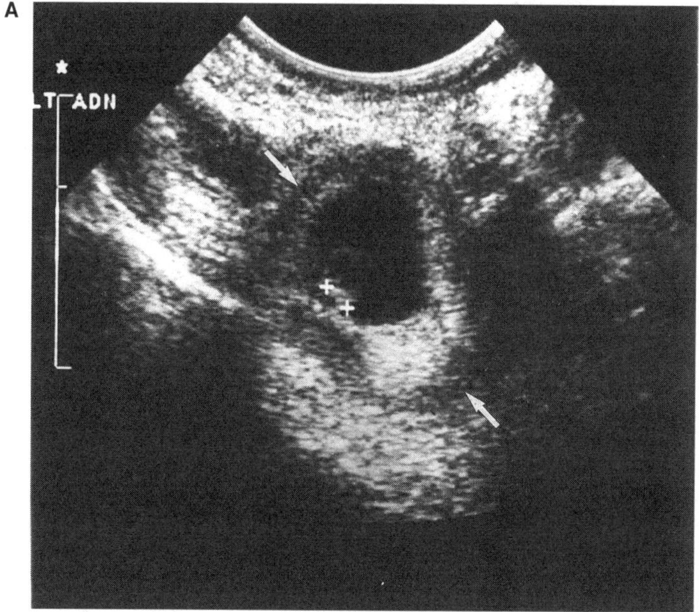

FIG. 4.19.

Persistent ectopic pregnancy. (A) On initial TVUS, an anechoic gestational sac (*arrows*) containing an embryo (*cursors*) is seen in the left adnexa. (B) The same patient as in part A. This patient presented with acute pelvic pain three weeks after undergoing laparoscopic salpingostomy for removal of previously demonstrated ectopic pregnancy. A large, disorganized, complex left adnexal mass (*arrows*) has developed, indicating recurrent trophoblastic tissue.

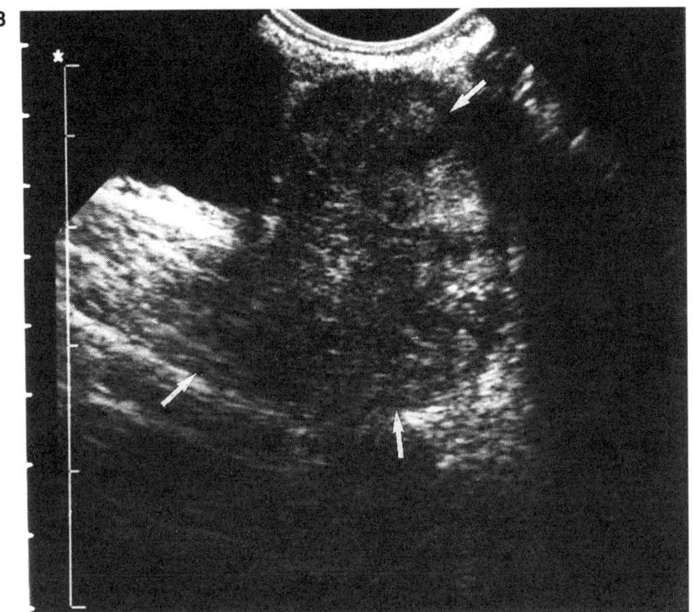

FIG. 4.19.

(*continued*).

recent reports as high as 1 per 2600 pregnancies (106–109). Patients undergoing assisted reproduction have an especially increased risk of heterotopic pregnancies.

A preoperative diagnosis is made in only 10% to 15% of all cases (107,110). Laboratory values, such as serum beta-hCG or progesterone, will be normal. When TVUS misses the diagnosis, the IUP alone is usually identified, and subsequent signs and symptoms may be falsely attributed to the IUP (110). Because the ectopic pregnancy is often diagnosed late, tubal rupture is common.

A high index of suspicion is necessary, especially in patients with known risk factors. The TVUS exam should comprise a deliberate, systematic assessment of the uterus and adnexae in all patients, regardless of clinical presentation or initial ultrasound findings.

Multiple Ectopic Pregnancies

More than 100 cases of multiple ectopic pregnancies have been reported, including both unilateral twins and bilateral ectopic pregnancies; this

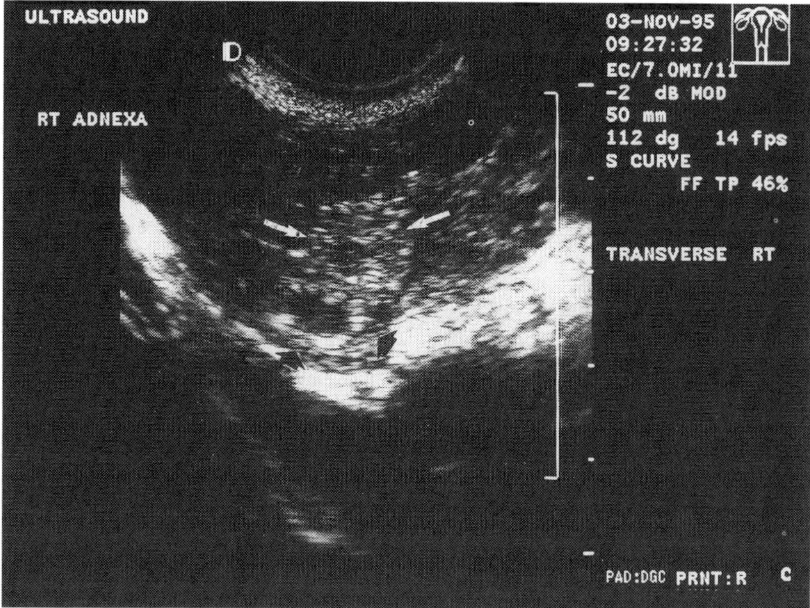

FIG. 4.20.

Twin tubal ectopic pregnancies. Two thick-walled, adjacent adnexal rings are visualized (*black arrows*). A yolk sac is present within one of the gestational sacs (*white arrows*).

type of pregnancy is more commonly reported with ultrasound than at pathology (Fig. 4.20) (111–113). The incidence of unilateral twins is likely higher than reported, because conservative surgery infrequently produces two intact gestational sacs for pathologic confirmation (113). Discrepancies in the size of multiple ectopic pregnancies are more likely related to difference in growth and viability, rather than metachronous origins.

NONTUBAL ECTOPIC PREGNANCIES

Interstitial Pregnancy

An interstitial pregnancy occurs after gestational sac implantation into the interstitial portion of the fallopian tube. This source accounts for 2% to 3% of all ectopic pregnancies (114,115). The vascular nature

TABLE 4.7

Interstitial Pregnancy — TVUS Signs

Eccentric gestational sac or complex mass, contiguous with the uterus

Myometrial thinning

Intrauterine gestational sac separate from the endometrial echo

Extension of the interstitial line to the gestational sac or complex mass

Manual ballottement of uterus during TVUS exam: an interstitial pregnancy should
move in unison with the uterus

Peripheral vascular flow on color/power Doppler

---

of the interstitial region of the uterus may cause severe hemorrhage following rupture, which usually occurs at a later gestational age than a tubal pregnancy (116–118). A live birth is not uncommon in this very distensible locale.

Table 4.7 details TVUS signs of interstitial pregnancy. TVUS examination will reveal an eccentric gestational sac or complex mass in the superolateral aspect of the uterus (Fig. 4.21). As these pregnancies are located in the extreme periphery of the uterus, the fundal and lateral uterine margins must be fully assessed in all patients.

The ectopic gestation is completely surrounded by myometrium and should be clearly separable from the endometrial echo (114,117). Myometrial thinning (less than 5 mm) is most commonly seen with an advanced intact gestational sac, but is an insensitive sign (114). An imperceptibly thin myometrial wall signals imminent rupture, and a surgeon should be notified immediately.

Ackerman reported the TVUS findings in 12 patients with an interstitial pregnancy (114). A thin linear interstitial line, representing the interstitial portion of the fallopian tube, was identified within the superolateral uterus (Fig. 4.22). The interstitial line should extend directly to the center of an interstitial gestational sac or complex mass, a sign that was 80% sensitive and 98% specific for an interstitial pregnancy. Eccentric gestational sac location (sensitivity = 40%, specificity = 88%) and myometrial thinning (sensitivity = 40%, specificity = 93%) were less

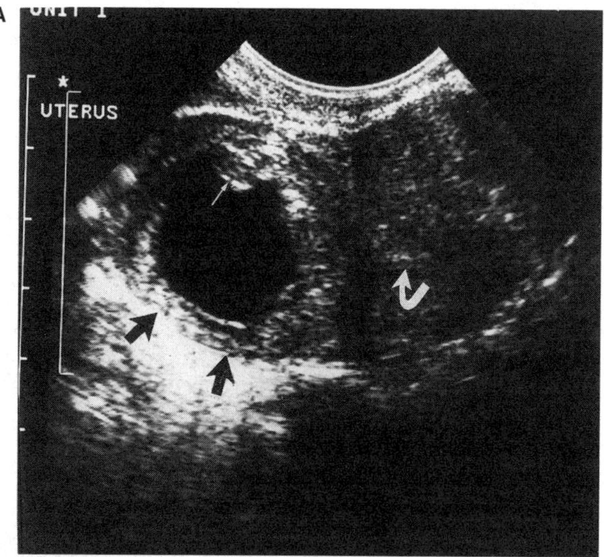

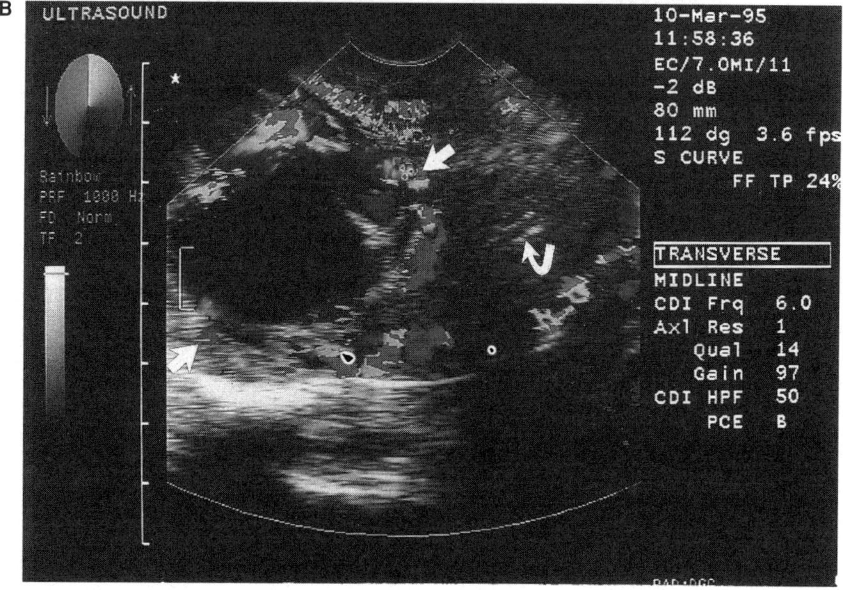

FIG. 4.21.

Interstitial ectopic pregnancy. (A) An eccentric gestational sac is laterally positioned within the uterus, causing myometrial thinning (*black arrows*). The gestational sac is separate from the endometrium (*curved arrow*) (*thin arrow* = nonviable embryo). (B) Exuberant color Doppler flow surrounds the gestational sac (*arrow* = peritrophoblastic flow, *curved arrow* = endometrium).

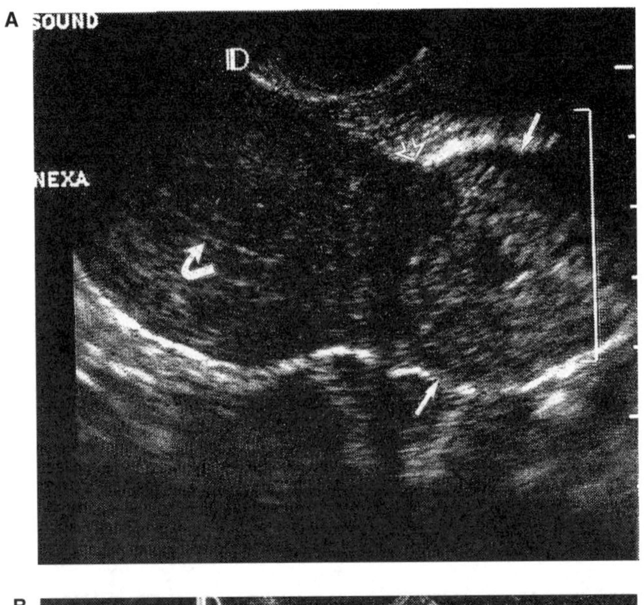
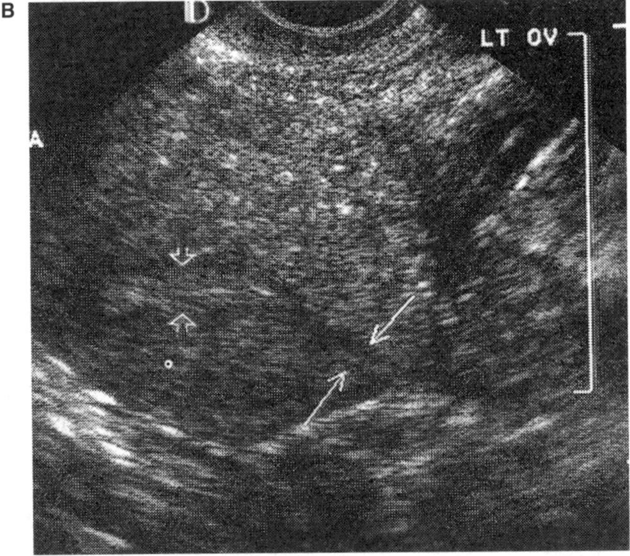

FIG. 4.22.

Interstitial line. (A) A hyperechoic mass (*solid arrows*) contiguous with left lateral uterine margin (*open arrow*) is considered suspicious for interstitial pregnancy (*curved arrow* = endometrium). (B) The same patient as in part B, with the image obtained at a slightly more inferior level. The interstitial line (*arrows*) is visualized in continuity with the endometrium (*open arrows*) and does not intersect the ectopic mass, excluding an interstitial pregnancy. An isthmic pregnancy was surgically confirmed.

reliable findings, although a correct diagnosis is nevertheless achievable using a combination of these signs (114).

Cervical Pregnancy

Cervical pregnancies account for 0.15% of all ectopic pregnancies (119). The predisposing factors adversely affect intrauterine implantation (IUD, prior dilatation and curettage or cesarean section, endometritis, leiomyomas, and Asherman's syndrome).

Table 4.8 lists the TVUS signs of cervical pregnancy. TVUS demonstrates a gestational sac or complex mass that has entirely developed within the cervix (Fig. 4.23). No fetal parts should be visible in the uterine cavity. A bulbous cervical contour occurs with growth, producing an hourglass configuration (120,121). An overdistended urinary bladder during a TAS may efface and obscure the cervical gestational sac or bulbous contour (121). Concerns that TVUS may dislodge or traumatize the cervical ectopic, provoking spontaneous hemorrhage, appear unfounded (119).

An inevitable abortion, necrotic cervical neoplasm, or complicated nabothian cyst can mimic the TVUS appearance of a cervical pregnancy. The presence of a live embryo within a cervical gestational sac confirms a cervical pregnancy; otherwise, a spontaneous inevitable abortion may have an identical TVUS appearance (120). It is critical to make a preoperative distinction between these two entities, because an inevitable abortion will, at worst, require a surgical evacuation. A surgical evacuation performed on a cervical pregnancy is contraindicated and may cause severe hemorrhage

---

TABLE 4.8

Cervical Ectopic Pregnancy — TVUS Signs

Bulbous cervix (hourglass sign)

Gestational sac completely within the cervix

Live embryo within intracervical sac

Increased Doppler flow surrounding cervical gestational sac

Thin endometrium

Absent peritrophoblastic Doppler arterial flow adjacent to endometrium

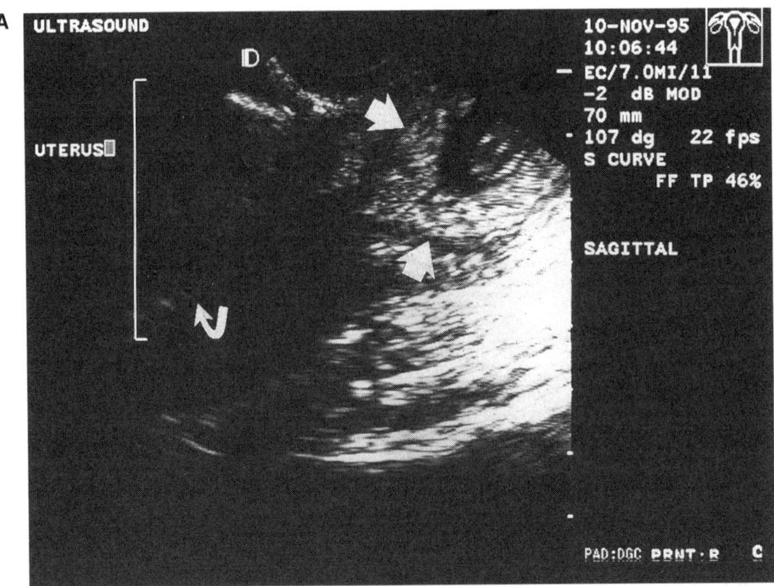

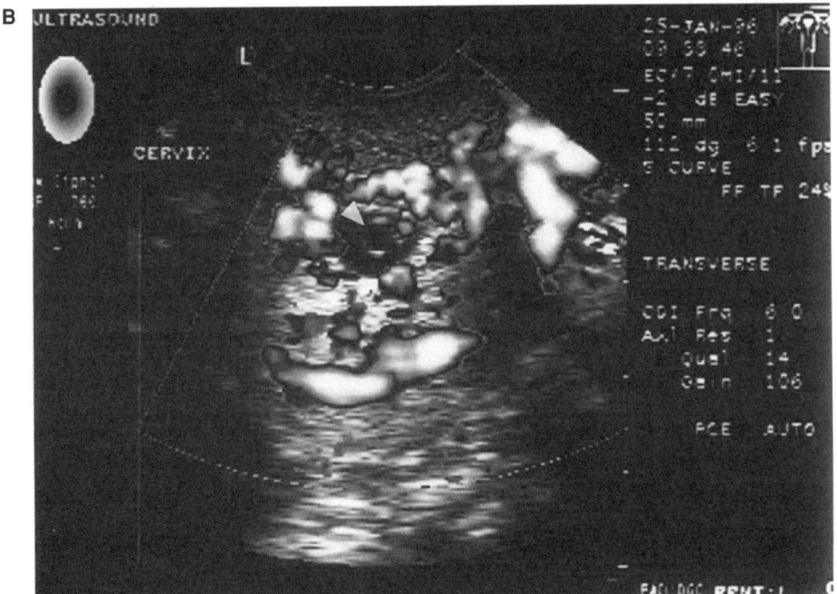

FIG. 4.23.

Cervical ectopic pregnancy. (A) TVUS of uterus in long-axis view. The thick-walled gestational sac appears within the cervix (*arrows*). Note the thin, linear endometrial echo (*curved arrow*). (B) Circumferential vascularity surrounding the cervical gestational sac on power Doppler (*arrowhead* = yolk sac).

(120). An inevitable abortion represents sloughing of a normally implanted intrauterine gestational sac first into the uterine and then into the cervical canal.

TVUS Doppler features are especially useful in distinguishing a cervical pregnancy from an inevitable abortion. A characteristic peritrophoblastic flow will surround the gestational sac of a cervical pregnancy (see Fig. 4.23B). An aborting gestational sac will lack adjacent low-impedance arterial flow within the cervix, and peritrophoblastic flow will be present adjacent to the original endometrial implantation site (Fig. 4.24) (123). TVUS has an overall high accuracy for the diagnosis of a cervical ectopic pregnancy.

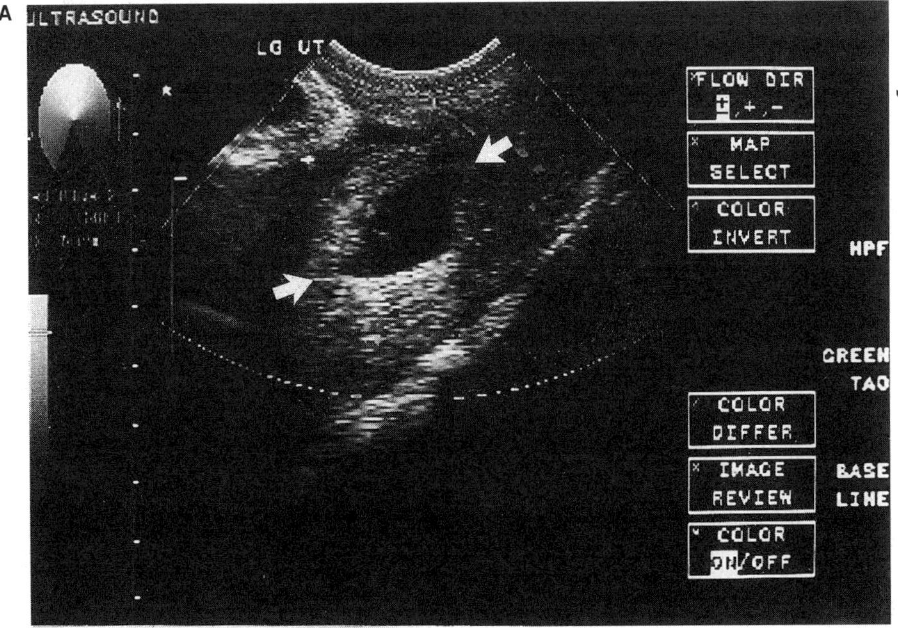

FIG. 4.24.

Cervical pregnancy versus inevitable abortion. (A) An intact gestational sac (*arrows*) is seen within the cervix. A lack of Doppler vascular flow suggests a nonviable cervical pregnancy. (B) Peritrophoblastic uterine flow upon TVUS of uterus. A focal area of low-resistance arterial flow is found adjacent to the endometrium (*arrow*), indicating the original implantation site. The gestational sac (*curved arrow*) represents an aborting gestational sac or an inevitable abortion.

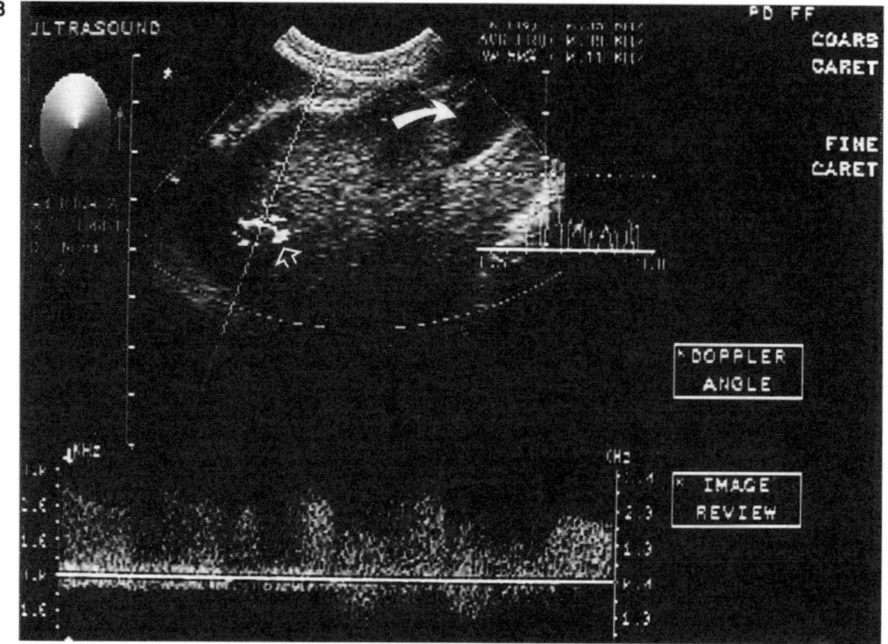

FIG. 4.24.

(*continued*).

The treatment of choice for cervical pregnancy is TVUS-guided aspiration of the conception products with injection of KCl into the gestational sac. Frates studied six cases successfully treated with local KCl injection, noting a gradual involution of the gestational sac following the procedure (119). Persistent complex material within the cervical canal can be visualized for as long as eight weeks after injection (Fig. 4.25).

Persistent hypervascularity surrounding an ablated cervical gestation has occurred despite adequate clinical responses. TVUS monitoring of such patients following ablation appears to be unnecessary and may even prove potentially confusing or misleading.

ABDOMINAL PREGNANCY

Stanley reviewed a series of 20 abdominal pregnancies in which a correct diagnosis was made in 15 cases (75%) (124). The most common and reliable

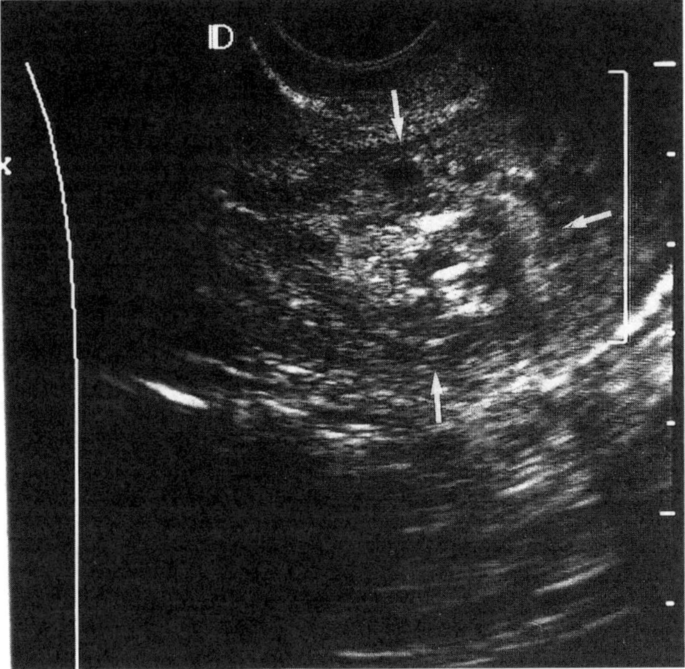

FIG. **4.25.**

TVUS of postablation cervical pregnancy. The same patient as Figure 4.23, two weeks after TVUS-guided KCl injection into the cervical gestational sac. A complex, disorganized mass (*arrows*) persists within the cervix.

sonographic finding was clear separation of the fetus from the uterus, which was seen retrospectively in 90% of cases. Scanning anteriorly with a high-frequency transducer will help to detect or rule out myometrium interposed between the amniotic cavity and maternal abdominal wall (Fig. 4.26).

Abdominal pregnancies are usually located cephalad to the uterus and may implant directly on the fundus of the small, nongravid uterus, an appearance that may simulate a cervix covered by placenta (pseudoprevia). When abdominal pregnancies advance into the second or third trimester, they are primarily evaluated with TAS. Recognizing the small uterus, empty uterine cavity, and low fundal position will be difficult without performing a complementary TVUS exam. Table 4.9 lists the TVUS signs of abdominal pregnancy.

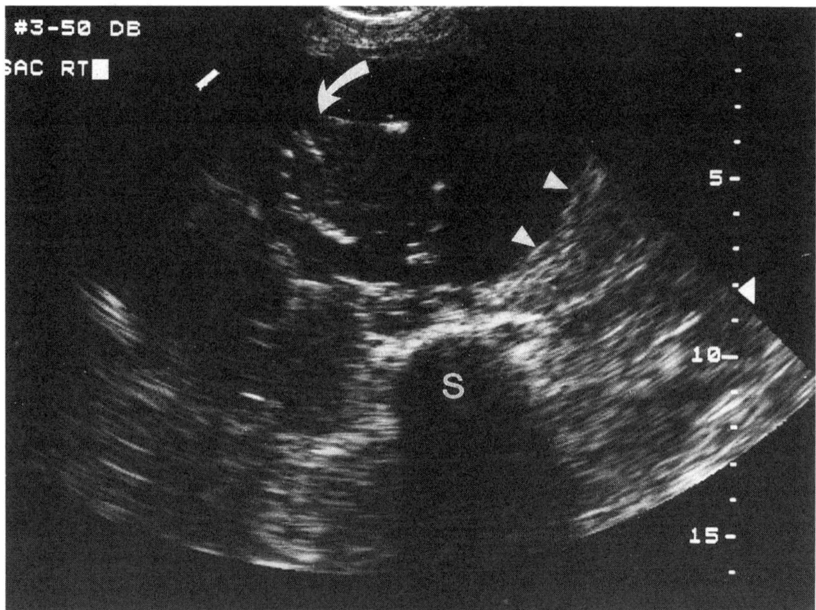

FIG. 4.26.

Abdominal pregnancy. TAS shows an 18-week-size pregnancy located in the upper pelvis (*curved arrow* = fetus, *s* = lumbar sign). The gestational sac wall is imperceptibly thin, without any surrounding myometrium (*arrowheads*).

TABLE 4.9

Abdominal Pregnancy — TVUS Signs

Fetus separate from uterine cavity

Gestational sac implanted on uterine fundus (pseudoprevia)

Low fundal position

Extrauterine placenta

Nonvisualized placenta

Nonvisualized myometrium surrounding gestational sac

Oligohydramnios

Maternal intraperitoneal fluid

Congenital deformities (club foot, Potter's facies)

Fetus too close to maternal abdominal wall

Fetus obscured by maternal bowel gas

An extrauterine placenta has been visualized in 75% of abdominal pregnancies. In 15% of cases, placental tissue was not identified, as it may be multifocal with implantation on various peritoneal surfaces (124,125). Oligohydramnios was reported in half of all cases, presumably resulting from absorption of amniotic fluid by the peritoneum (124,126). Congenital deformations associated with severe oligohydramnios are common as well. Maternal free intraperitoneal fluid was present in 10% of patients.

An extrauterine fetus located within the cul-de-sac may result from an abdominal pregnancy, ovarian pregnancy, or a ruptured tubal or intrauterine pregnancy (Fig. 4.27) (127). Careful attention to sonographic criteria should enable a correct diagnosis in 90% of cases (124).

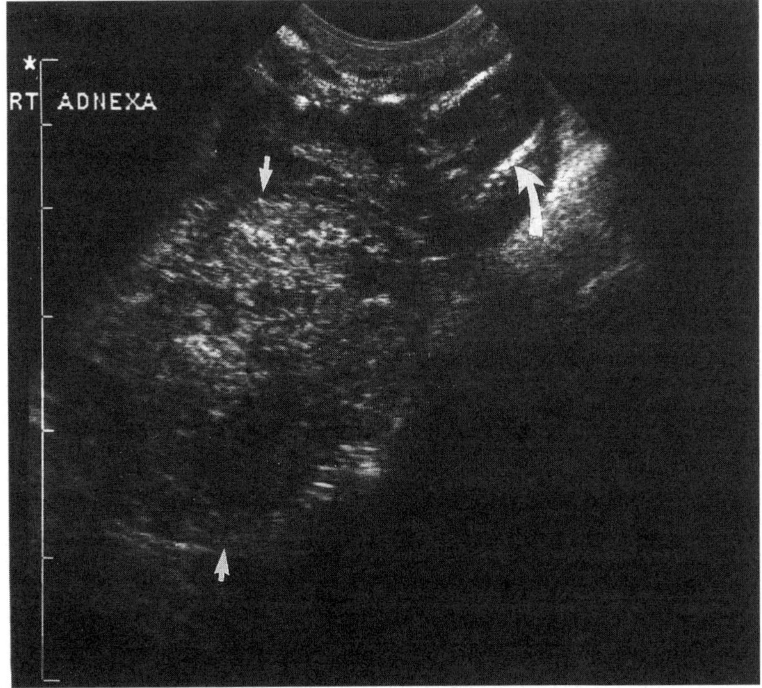

FIG. 4.27.

Fetus in cul-de-sac. A 12-week-size fetus (*curved arrow*) and hyperechoic placental tissue (*short arrows*) are present within the cul-de-sac. These findings may occur with an abdominal or ovarian pregnancy, but take the form of an acutely ruptured tubal pregnancy in this patient.

OVARIAN PREGNANCY

Ovarian pregnancy is very rare, accounting for less than 1% of all ectopic pregnancies (126,128). Trophoblastic invasion into the highly vascular ovary frequently results in early hemorrhage and rupture, and patients present early in gestation with adnexal pain or hemoperitoneum (116). The clinical, sonographic, and surgical appearance of an ovarian pregnancy closely impersonates the appearance of a hemorrhagic or ruptured corpus luteum cyst (128). Accurate preoperative and intraoperative diagnosis is difficult, with Hallock reporting a correct surgical diagnosis in only 28% of cases (129).

An ovarian pregnancy commonly appears as a complex mass, with surrounding echogenic cul-de-sac fluid and a nonvisualized ipsilateral ovary (Fig. 4.28) (130). TVUS may identify an intraovarian gestational sac

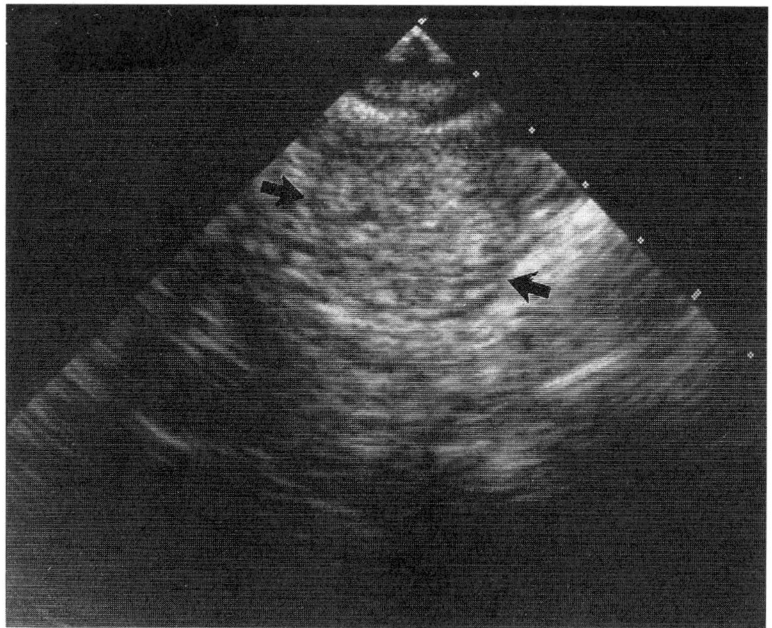

FIG. 4.28.

Ovarian pregnancy. Round, hyperechoic, adnexal mass (*arrows*). The ipsilateral ovary was not sonographically identified. Diagnosis of ovarian pregnancy made only after histologic examination of a surgical specimen.

TABLE 4.10

Ovarian Pregnancy — TVUS Signs

Intraovarian gestational sac
  Live embryo within ovary
Complex adnexal mass with nonvisualization of the ipsilateral ovary
Hemoperitoneum

(Table 4.10), but the diagnosis is both uncommon and difficult without visualization of an embryo (128). An intraovarian gestational sac and a corpus luteum may both present as a hyperechoic, thick-walled, cystic mass with low-impedance arterial circumferential flow on color Doppler. Pathologic confirmation is also impaired when conservative surgery, along with early rupture, limits the volume and integrity of tissue available for analysis (129).

REFERENCES

1. Centers for Disease Control. Current trends: ectopic pregnancies — United States, 1979–1980. MMWR 1984;33:201–202.
2. Atrash HK, Friede A, Hogue CJ. Ectopic pregnancy mortality in the United States, 1970–1983. Obstet Gynecol 1987;70:817–822.
3. Centers for Disease Control. Ectopic pregnancies — United States, 1990–1992. MMWR 1995;44:46–48.
4. Chambers SE, Muir BB, Haddad NG. Ultrasound evaluation of ectopic pregnancy including correlation with human chorionic gonadotrophin levels. Br J Rad 1990;63:246–250.
5. Mattingly RL, Thompson JD. TeLinde's operative gynecology, 6th ed. Philadelphia: JB Lippincott, 1985:429–448.
6. Daus K, Mundy D, Graves W, Slade BA. Ectopic pregnancy: what to do during the 20-day window. J Reprod Med 1989;34:162–166.
7. Bonilla-Musoles FM, Ballester MJ, Tarin JJ, Raga F, Osborne NG, Pellicer A. Does transvaginal color Doppler sonography differentiate between developing and involuting ectopic pregnancies? J Ultrasound Med 1995;14:175–181.

8. Muller JE, Hacker J, Terinde R, Kozlowski P. Wandel von diagnostik und therapie der extrauteringraviditat mit besonderer bewertung des ultraschalls. Geburtsh Frauenheilk 1986;46:221–226.

9. Taylor KJ, Meyer WR. New techniques in the diagnosis of ectopic pregnancy. Obstet Gynecol Clin NA 1991;18:39–54.

10. Wojak JC, Clayton MJ, Nolan TE. Outcomes of ultrasound diagnosis of ectopic pregnancy: dependence on observer experience. Invest Rad 1995;30:115–117.

11. O'Brien MC, Rutherford T. Misdiagnosis of bilateral ectopic pregnancies: a caveat about operator expertise in the use of transvaginal ultrasound. J ER Med 1993;11:275–278.

12. Parvey HR, Maklad N. Pitfalls in the transvaginal sonographic diagnosis of ectopic pregnancy. J Ultrasound Med 1993;13:139–144.

13. Turetsky DB, Alexander AA, Linden SS. Pseudogestational sac of ectopic pregnancy simulating intrauterine pregnancy with transvaginal sonography. J Clin Ultrasound 1991;19:120–123.

14. Crade M. Transvaginal imaging of ectopic pregnancy. Western J Med 1991;155:3.

15. Serafini P, Batzofin J. Transvaginal color Doppler ultrasonography in reproductive gynecology. Int J Fertil 1994;39:253–261.

16. Rempen A. Vaginal sonography in ectopic pregnancy: a prospective evaluation. J Ultrasound Med 1988;7:381–387.

17. Myberg DA, Mack LA, Jeffrey RB Jr, Laing FC. Endovaginal sonographic evaluation of ectopic pregnancy: a prospective study. AJR Am J Roentgenol 1987;149:1181–1186.

18. Alfirevic Z, Kurjak A. Transvaginal colour Doppler ultrasound in normal and abnormal early pregnancy. J Perinat Med 1990;18:173–180.

19. Rubin JM. Power Doppler ultrasound: a potentially useful alternative to mean frequency-based color ultrasound. Radiology 1994;190:853–856.

20. Taylor KJ, Burns PN, Woodcock JP, et al. Blood flow in deep abdominal and pelvic vessels: ultrasonic pulsed-Doppler analysis. Radiology 1985;154:487–493.

21. Thompson RS, Trudinger BJ, Cook CM. Doppler ultrasound waveform indices: A/B ratio, pulsatility index and Pourcelot ratio. Br J Obstet Gynaecol 1988;95:581–588.

22. Daya S, Woods S, Ward S, Lappalainen R, Caco C. Transvaginal ultrasound scanning in early pregnancy and correlation with human chorionic gonadotropin levels. J Clin Ultrasound 1991;19:139–142.

23. Kadar N, Devore G, Romero R. Discriminatory hCG zone: its use in the sonographic evaluation for ectopic pregnancy. Obstet Gynecol 1981;58:156–160.
24. Peisner DB, Timor-Tritsch IE. The discriminatory zone of beta-hCG for vaginal probes. J Clin Ultrasound 1990;18:280–285.
25. Bernaschek G, Rudelstorfer R, Csaicsich P. Vaginal sonography versus serum human gonadotropin in early detection of pregnancy. Am J Obstet Gynecol 1988;158:608–612.
26. Bocciolone L, Vercellini P, Villa L, Rognoni MT, Dorta M, Fedele L. Early detection of ectopic pregnancy: use of a sensitive urine pregnancy test and transvaginal sonography. J Reprod Med 1991;36:496–499.
27. Shapiro BS, Cullen M, Taylor KJ, DeCherney AH. Transvaginal ultrasonography for the diagnosis of ectopic pregnancy. Fertil Steril 1988;50:425–429.
28. Romero R, Kadar N, Jeanty P. Diagnosis of ectopic pregnancy: value of the discriminatory human chorionic gonadotropin zone. Obstet Gynecol 1985;66:357–360.
29. Stiller RJ, Haynes de Regt R, Blair E. Transvaginal ultrasonography in patients at risk for ectopic pregnancy. Am J Obstet Gynecol 1989;161:930–933.
30. de Crespigny LCh. Demonstration of ectopic pregnancy by transvaginal ultrasound. Br J Obstet Gynecol 1988;95:1253–1256.
31. Kurjak A, Zalud I, Schulman H. Ectopic pregnancy: transvaginal color Doppler of trophoblastic flow in questionable adnexa. J Ultrasound Med 1991;10:685–689.
32. van Dam PA, Vanderheyden JS, Uyttenbroeck F. Application of ultrasound in the diagnosis of heterotopic pregnancy—a review of the literature. J Clin Ultrasound 1988;16:159–165.
33. Achiron R, Goldenberg M, Lipitz S, Mashiach S, Oelsner G. Transvaginal Doppler sonography for detecting ectopic pregnancy: is it really necessary? Isr J Med Sci 1994;30:820–825.
34. Schurz B, Wenzl R, Eppel W, Schon HJ, Reinold E. Early detection of ectopic pregnancy by transvaginal ultrasound. Arch Gynecol Obstet 1990;248:25–29.
35. Timor-Tritsch IE, Yeh M, Peisner DB, Lesser KB, Slavik TA. The use of transvaginal sonography in the diagnosis of ectopic pregnancy. Am J Obstet Gynecol 1989;161:157–161.
36. Taylor RN. Ectopic pregnancy and reproductive technology. JAMA 1988;259:1862–1864.

37. Abramovici H, Auslender R, Lewin A, et al. Gestational-pseudogestational sac. A new ultrasonic criterion for differential diagnosis. Am J Obstet Gynecol 1983;145:377–379.
38. Nyberg DA, Laing FC, Filly RA, Uri-Simmons M, Jeffrey RB. Ultrasonographic differentiation of the gestational sac of early intrauterine pregnancy for the pseudogestational sac of ectopic pregnancy. Radiology 1983;146:755–759.
39. Ackerman TE, Levi CS, Lyons EA, Dashefsky SM, Lindsay DJ, Holt SC. Decidual cyst: endovaginal sonographic sign of ectopic pregnancy. Radiology 1993;189:727–731.
40. Bradley WG, Fiske CE, Filly RA. The double sac sign of early intrauterine pregnancy: use in exclusion of ectopic pregnancy. Radiology 1982;143:223–226.
41. Jain KA, Hamper UM, Sanders RC. Comparison of transvaginal and transabdominal sonography in the detection of early pregnancy and its complications. AJR Am J Roentgenol 1988;151:1139–1143.
42. Nyberg DA, Laing FC, Filly RA. Threatened abortion: sonographic distinction of normal and abnormal sacs. Radiology 1986;158:397–400.
43. Nyberg DA, Mack LA, Harvey D, Wang K. Value of the yolk sac in evaluating early pregnancies. J Ultrasound Med 1988;7:129–135.
44. Dillon EH, Feyock AL, Taylor KJ. Pseudogestational sacs: Doppler US differentiation from normal or abnormal intrauterine pregnancies. Radiology 1990;176:359–364.
45. Taylor KJ, Ramos IM, Feyock AL, et al. Ectopic pregnancy: duplex Doppler evaluation. Radiology 1989;173:93–97.
46. Kurjak A, Crvenkovic G, Salihagic A, Zalud I, Miljan M. The assessment of normal early pregnancy by transvaginal color Doppler sonography. J Clin Ultrasound 1993;21:3–8.
47. Emerson DS, Cartier MS, Altieri LA. Diagnostic efficacy on endovaginal color Doppler flow imaging in an ectopic pregnancy screening program. Radiology 1992;183:413–420.
48. Kurtz AB, Shlansky-Goldberg RD, Choi HY, Needleman L, Wapner RJ, Goldberg BB. Detection of retained products of conception following spontaneous abortion in the first trimester. J Ultrasound Med 1991;10:387–395.
49. Pellerito JS, Taylor KJ. Ectopic pregnancy: evaluation with endovaginal color Doppler flow imaging — response. Radiology 1993;187:21–22.
50. Achiron R, Goldenberg M, Lipitz S, Mashiach S. Transvaginal duplex Doppler ultrasonography in bleeding patients suspected of having residual trophoblastic tissue. Obstet Gynecol 1993;81:507–511.

51. Dillon EH, Case CQ, Ramos IM, Holland CK, Taylor KJ. Endovaginal US and Doppler findings after first-trimester abortion. Radiology 1993;186:87–91.

52. Miller DL. Update on safety of diagnostic ultrasonography. J Clin Ultrasound 1991;19:531–540.

53. Coleman BG, Baron RL, Arger PH. Ectopic embryo detection using real-time sonography. J Clin Ultrasound 1985;13:545–554.

54. Lopez HB, Micheelsen U, Berendtsen H, Kock K. Ectopic pregnancy and its associated changes. Gynecol Obstet Invest 1994;38:104–106.

55. Enk L, Wikland M, Hammarberg K, Lindblom B. The value of endovaginal sonography and urinary human chorionic gonadotropin tests for the differentiation between intrauterine and ectopic pregnancy. J Clin Ultrasound 1990;18:73–78.

56. Atri M, de Stempel J, Bret PM. Accuracy of transvaginal ultrasonography for detection of hematosalpinx in ectopic pregnancy. J Clin Ultrasound 1992;20:255–261.

57. Hill LM, Kislak S, Martin JG. Transvaginal sonographic detection of the pseudogestational sac associated with ectopic pregnancy. Obstet Gynecol 1990;75:986–988.

58. Jurkovic D, Bourne TH, Jauniaux E, Campbell S, Collins WP. Transvaginal color Doppler study of blood flow in ectopic pregnancies. Fertil Steril 1992;57:68–73.

59. Parsons AK. Ultrasound of the human corpus luteum. Ultrasound Quarterly 1994;12:127–166.

60. Dillon EH, Taylor KJ. Doppler ultrasound in the female pelvis and first trimester of pregnancy. Clin Diagn Ultrasound 1990;26:99–107.

61. Taylor KJ, Burns PN, Conway DL, Hull MG. Ultrasound Doppler flow studies of the ovarian and uterine arteries. Br J Obstet Gynecol 1985;92:240–246.

62. Salim A, Zalud I, Farmakides G, Schulman H, Kurjak A, Latin V. Corpus luteum blood flow in normal and abnormal pregnancy: evaluation with transvaginal color and pulsed Doppler sonography. J Ultrasound Med 1994;13:971–975.

63. Walters MD, Eddy C, Pauerstein CJ. The contralateral corpus luteum and tubal pregnancy. Obstet Gynecol 1987;70:823–826.

64. Pellerito JS, Taylor KJ, Quedens-Case C. Ectopic pregnancy: evaluation with endovaginal color flow imaging. Radiology 1992;183:407–411.

65. Gjelland K, Hordnes K, Tjugum J, Augensen K, Bergsjo P. Treatment of ectopic pregnancy by local injection of hypertonic glucose: a randomized

trial comparing administration guided by transvaginal ultrasound or laparoscopy. Acta Obstet Gynecol Scand 1995;74:629–634.

66. Hess LW, Peaceman A, O'Brien WF, Winkel CA, Cruikshank DP, Morrison JC. Adnexal mass occurring with intrauterine pregnancy: report of fifty-four patients requiring laparotomy for definitive management. Am J Obstet Gynecol 1988;158:1029–1034.

67. Brown DL, Doubilet PM. Transvaginal sonography for diagnosing ectopic pregnancy: positivity criteria and performance characteristics. J Ultrasound Med 1994;13:259–266.

68. Kooi S, Kock HC. Treatment of tubal pregnancy by local injection of methotrexate after adrenaline injection into the mesosalpinx: a report of 25 patients. Fertil Steril 1990;54:580–584.

69. Tulandi T, Bret PM, Atri M, Senterman M. Treatment of ectopic pregnancy by transvaginal intratubal methotrexate administration. Obstet Gynecol 1991;77:627–630.

70. Stovall TG, Ling FW. Single-dose methotrexate: an expanded clinical trial. Am J Obstet Gynecol 1993;168:1759–1765.

71. Tekay A, Martikainen H, Heikkinen H, Kivela A, Jouppila P. Disappearance of the trophoblastic blood flow in tubal pregnancy after methotrexate injection. J Ultrasound Med 1993;12:615–618.

72. Atri M, Bret PM, Tulandi T, Senterman MK. Ectopic pregnancy: evolution after treatment with transvaginal methotrexate. Radiology 1992;185:749–753.

73. Fleischer AC, Pennell RG, McKee MS. Ectopic pregnancy: features at transvaginal sonography. Radiology 1990;174:375–378.

74. Tongsong T, Pongsatha S. Transvaginal sonographic features in diagnosis of ectopic pregnancy. Int J Gynecol Obstet 1993;43:277–283.

75. Cacciatore B. Can the status of tubal pregnancy be predicted with transvaginal sonography? A prospective comparison of sonographic, surgical, and serum hCG findings. Radiology 1990;177:481–484.

76. Caspi E, Sherman D. Tubal abortion and infundibular ectopic pregnancy. Clin Obstet Gynecol 1987;30:155–163.

77. Tekay A, Jouppila P. Color Doppler flow as an indicator of trophoblastic activity in tubal pregnancies detected by transvaginal ultrasound. Obstet Gynecol 1992;80:995–999.

78. Thorsen MK, Lawson TL, Aiman EJ, et al. Diagnosis of ectopic pregnancy: endovaginal vs transabdominal sonography. AJR Am J Roentgenol 1990;155:307–310.

79. Meyer WR, DeCherney AH, Diamond MP. Tubal ectopic pregnancy: contemporary diagnosis, treatment, and reproductive potential. J Gynecol Surg 1989;5:343–352.

80. Timor-Tritsch IE. Vaginal sonography in the diagnosis of ectopic pregnancy (letter, reply). Am J Obstet Gynecol 1990;162:1640–1641.

81. Dashefsky SM, Lyons EA, Levi CS, Lindsay DJ. Suspected ectopic pregnancy: endovaginal and transvesical US. Radiology 1988;169:181–184.

82. Laing FC. Sonographic determination of tubal rupture in patients with ectopic pregnancy: is it feasible? Radiology 1990;177:330–331.

83. Nyberg DA, Hughes MP, Mack LA, Wang KY. Extrauterine findings of ectopic pregnancy at transvaginal US: importance of echogenic fluid. Radiology 1991;178:823–836.

84. Sadek AL, Schiotz HA. Transvaginal sonography in the management of ectopic pregnancy. Acta Obstet Gynecol Scand 1995;74:293–296.

85. Nyberg DA, Mack LA, Laing FC, Jeffrey RB. Early pregnancy complications: endovaginal sonographic findings correlated with human chorionic gonadotropin levels. Radiology 1988;167:619–622.

86. Subramanyam BR, Raghavendra BN, Balthazar EJ, Horii SC, Hilton S, Goldstein SR. Hematosalpinx in tubal pregnancy: sonographic-pathologic correlation. AJR 1983;141:361–365.

87. Meyers MA. Dynamic radiology of the abdomen: normal and abnormal anatomy, 3rd ed. New York: Springer-Verlag, 1988:49–71.

88. Ankum WM, Van der Veen F, Hamerlynck JV, Lammes FB. Suspected ectopic pregnancy: what to do when human chorionic gonadotropin levels are below the discriminatory zone. J Reprod Med 1995;40: 525–528.

89. Hahlin M, Thorburn J, Bryman I. The expectant management of early pregnancies of uncertain site. Hum Reprod 1995;10:1223–1227.

90. Stabile I, Grudzinskas J, Campbell S. Doppler ultrasonographic evaluation of abnormal pregnancies in the first trimester. J Clin Ultrasound 1990;18:497–501.

91. Cacciatore B, Korhonen J, Stenman UH, Ylostalo P. Transvaginal sonography and serum hCG in monitoring of presumed ectopic pregnancies selected for expectant management. Ultrasound Obstet Gynecol 1995;5: 297–300.

92. Brown DL. Diagnosis of ectopic pregnancy with endovaginal color Doppler US. Radiology 1993;187:20.

93. Atri M. Ectopic pregnancy: evaluation with endovaginal color Doppler flow imaging. Radiology 1993;187:19.

94. Frates MC, Brown DL, Doubilet PM, Hornstein MD. Tubal rupture in patients with ectopic pregnancy: diagnosis with transvaginal US. Radiology 1994;191:769–772.

95. Ylostalo P, Cacciatore B, Sjoberg J, Kaariainen M, Tenhunen A, Stenman UH. Expectant management of ectopic pregnancy. Obstet Gynecol 1992;80:345–348.

96. Wolf GC, Nickisch SA, George KE, Teicher JR, Simms TD. Completely nonsurgical management of ectopic pregnancies. Gynecol Obstet Invest 1994;37:232–235.

97. Cacciatore B, Stenman UH, Ylostalo P. Early screening for ectopic pregnancy in high-risk symptom-free women. Lancet 1994;343:517–518.

98. Timor-Tritsch I, Baxi L, Peisner DB. Transvaginal salpingocentesis: a new technique for treating ectopic pregnancy. Am J Obstet Gynecol 1989;160:459–461.

99. Fernandez H, Rainhorn JD, Papiernik E, Bellet D, Frydman R. Spontaneous resolution of ectopic pregnancy. Obstet Gynecol 1988;71:171–174.

100. Menard A, Crequat J, Mandelbrot L, Hauuy J, Madelenat P. Treatment of unruptured tubal pregnancy by local injection of methotrexate under transvaginal sonographic control. Fertil Steril 1990;54:47–50.

101. Tulandi T, Hemmings R, Khalifa F. Rupture of ectopic pregnancy in women with low and declining serum beta-human chorionic gonadotropin concentrations. Fertil Steril 1991;56:786–787.

102. Atri M, Bret PM, Tulandi T. Spontaneous resolution of ectopic pregnancy: initial appearance and evolution at transvaginal US. Radiology 1993;186:83–86.

103. Kuo D, Chiu T, Hsieh T, Soong Y. Serial sonographic changes in a case of isthmic pregnancy treated with methotrexate. J Clin Ultrasound 1993;21:460–463.

104. Seifer DB, Diamond MP, DeCherney AH. Persistent ectopic pregnancy. Obstet Gynecol Clin NA 1991;18:153–159.

105. Parker J, Thompson D. Persistent ectopic pregnancy after conservative management: successful treatment with single-dose intramuscular methotrexate. Aust NZ J Obstet Gynecol 1994;34:99–102.

106. Richards S, Stempel L, Carlton B. Heterotopic pregnancy: reappraisal of incidence. Am J Obstet Gynecol 1982;142:928–930.

107. Rizk B, Seang LT, Morcos S, et al. Heterotopic pregnancies after in vitro fertilization and embryo transfer. Am J Obstet Gynecol 1991;164:161–164.

108. Reece EA, Petrie RH, Sirmans MF, et al. Combined intrauterine and extrauterine gestations: a review. Am J Obstet Gynecol 1983;146:323–330.

109. Hann LE, Bachman DM, McArdle CR. Coexistent intrauterine and ectopic pregnancy: a reevaluation. Radiology 1984;152:151–154.

110. Wong WS, Mao K. Combined intrauterine and tubal ectopic pregnancy. Aust NZ J Obstet Gynecol 1989;29:76–77.

111. Ash KM, Lyons EA, Levi CS, Lindsay DJ. Endovaginal sonographic diagnosis of ectopic twin gestation. J Ultrasound Med 1991;10:497–500.

112. Sherer DM, Liberto L, Woods JR. Preoperative sonographic diagnosis of a unilateral tubal twin gestation with documented fetal heart activity. J Ultrasound Med 1990;9:729–731.

113. Gerscovich EO, McGahan JP. High-resolution ultrasonography in the diagnosis of twin tubal ectopic pregnancies. J Clin Ultrasound 1991;19:501–504.

114. Ackerman TE, Levi CS, Dashefsky SM, Holt SC, Lindsay DJ. Interstitial line: sonographic finding in interstitial (cornual) ectopic pregnancy. Radiology 1993;189:83–87.

115. Chen G, Lin M, Lee M. Diagnosis of interstitial pregnancy with sonography. J Clin Ultrasound 1994;22:439–442.

116. Bayless RB. Nontubal ectopic pregnancy. Clin Obstet Gynecol 1987;30:191–199.

117. Sherer DM, Allen T, Singh GS, Woods JR. Transvaginal sonographic diagnosis of unruptured interstitial pregnancy. J Clin Ultrasound 1990;18:582–585.

118. Confino E, Gleicher N. Conservative surgical management of interstitial pregnancy. Fertil Steril 1989;52:600–603.

119. Frates MC, Benson CB, Doubilet PM, et al. Cervical ectopic pregnancy: results of conservative treatment. Radiology 1994;191:773–775.

120. Sherer DM, Abramowicz JS, Thompson HO, Liberto L, Angel C, Woods JR. Comparison of transabdominal and endovaginal sonographic approaches in the diagnosis of a case of cervical pregnancy successfully treated with methotrexate. J Ultrasound Med 1991;10:409–411.

121. Centini G, Rosignoli L, Severi FM. A case of cervical pregnancy. Am J Obstet Gynecol 1994;171:272–273.

122. Armstrong B, Shah Y, Rubens D. Use of ultrasound and magnetic resonance imaging in the diagnosis of cervical pregnancy. J Clin Ultrasound 1989;17:283–286.

123. Rosenberg RD, Williamson MR. Cervical ectopic pregnancy: avoiding pitfalls in the ultrasonographic diagnosis. J Ultrasound Med 1992;11:365–367.

124. Stanley JH, Horger EO, Fagan CJ, Andriole JG, Fleischer A. Sonographic findings in abdominal pregnancy. AJR Am J Roentgenol 1986;147:1043–1046.

125. Costa SD, Presley J, Bastert G. Advanced abdominal pregnancy. Obstet Gynecol Survey 1991;46:515–525.
126. Athey PA, Jayson HT, Estrada R, Watson AB. Sonographic findings in primary ovarian pregnancy. J Clin Ultrasound 1990;18:730–732.
127. Gao J, Kazam E, Whalen J. Detection of the fetus in the cul-de-sac by transabdominal and transvaginal ultrasound: a case report. Clin Imaging 1991;15:296–298.
128. Belfar H, Heller K, Edelstone DI, Hill LM, Martin JG. Ovarian pregnancy resulting in a surviving neonate: ultrasound findings. J Ultrasound Med 1991;10:465–467.
129. Hallatt JG. Primary ovarian pregnancy: a report of twenty-five cases. Am J Obstet Gynecol 1982;143:55–58.
130. Maeyama M, Inoue S, Yoshikawa A, Tooya T, Iwamasa. A case of primary ovarian pregnancy. Acta Obstet Gynecol Scand 1985;64:363–366.
131. Ricci M, Mancini L, Santini D, De Jaco P, Orlandi C, Martinelli G. Primary ovarian pregnancy: a clinicopathologic study. Arch Anat Cytol Path 1988;36:108–111.

Systemic Methotrexate for Management of Ectopic Pregnancy

Thomas G. Stovall
John R. Brumsted

SYSTEMIC METHOTREXATE

The use of systemic methotrexate represents the single greatest advancement in the treatment of ectopic pregnancy since the introduction of surgery for the treatment of the condition. When it was first introduced, surgery was a life-saving surgical procedure. More recently, laparoscopic diagnosis and treatment have reduced to some extent the morbidity and cost associated with surgical therapy.

Since the inception of medical treatment for ectopic pregnancy, the goal has been to develop a completely nonsurgical approach to both diagnosis and treatment. Of equal importance, however, are the goals of developing a treatment regimen that is effective, associated with low toxicity, and able to preserve tubal function. If medical therapy is to gain widespread application, ideally it should be performed in a framework where laparoscopy is not required for diagnosis. Although this chapter does not focus on this development, a diagnostic algorithm that allows most patients to have the diagnosis of ectopic pregnancy confirmed without laparoscopy has been reported (1,2). It uses a combination of history and physical examination, risk factor assessment, urine pregnancy test, quantitative human chorionic gonadotropin (hCG), serum progesterone, transvaginal ultrasound with or without color Doppler, and suction curettage in selected patients with an abnormal pregnancy (3–7).

Although laparoscopy remains the gold standard for diagnosis of ectopic pregnancy, nonsurgical confirmation of this condition offers the advantages of decreased cost and avoidance of the risk of surgery and anesthesia. Eliminating laparoscopy also avoids the possibility of a false-negative or false-positive laparoscopic result.

PHARMACOLOGY OF METHOTREXATE

Gynecologists have vast experience with methotrexate treatment of gestational trophoblastic disease, and this therapy has been used extensively for this condition since 1956 (8). Methotrexate is a folic acid analogue that inhibits dehydrofolate reductase, thereby preventing synthesis of DNA; it has been shown to inhibit normal trophoblasts in vitro (9).

When methotrexate is administered in large doses or with prolonged treatment courses, side effects may occur. Commonly reported side effects include leukopenia, thrombocytopenia, bone marrow aplasia, ulcerative stomatitis, diarrhea, and hemorrhagic enteritis. Other reported side effects include alopecia, dermatitis, elevated liver enzymes, and pneumonitis (10,11). Citrovorum factor reduces the incidence of these unwanted effects and is generally used with patients undergoing prolonged treatment courses (12,13).

Importantly, long-term follow-up of women treated with methotrexate for gestational trophoblastic disease shows no increase in congenital malformation, spontaneous abortions, or second tumors after chemotherapy (14–16). Consequently, none would be expected after treatment of ectopic pregnancy, because a smaller total dose is required and shorter treatment duration is used in such cases.

PRIMARY TREATMENT

Methotrexate was first administered to treat an unruptured interstitial ectopic pregnancy using a 15-day intramuscular treatment regimen (17).

Subsequently, several investigators reported additional cases that in total described a very limited experience (18–21).

In 1986, Ory et al published their experience with six patients treated with 1.0 mg/kg intravenous methotrexate alternating with intramuscular citrovorum (0.2 mg/kg) for eight days. All patients underwent confirmatory laparoscopy pretreatment, and all had an unruptured ampullary ectopic pregnancy. Five of six patients (83.3%) were successfully treated. On the other hand, 50% of patients experienced a side effect, if one counts the two patients who required transfusion due to a falling hematocrit in this number (22).

Ichinoe et al (23) reported 23 patients with presumed ectopic pregnancies treated with 0.4 mg/kg/day intramuscular methotrexate for five days every other week until the hCG titer became negative. Of the 23 women treated, 22 (95.7%) responded successfully, with a mean resolution time of 29.7 days (range 6 to 47 days). None of the patients reported severe side effects, although minor side effects were noted in 20%.

In an effort to reduce the incidence of side effects, Sauer et al (24) treated 21 patients with a four-dose regimen using a combination of methotrexate and citrovorum following laparoscopic documentation of the unruptured ectopic pregnancy. Under this protocol, patients were treated with intramuscular methotrexate (1.0 mg/kg) on postoperative days 1, 3, 5, and 7, followed by administration of citrovorum factor (0.1 mg/kg) on days 2, 4, 6, and 8. Patients remained hospitalized until their hCG titer levels fell below their preoperative levels. Notably, 9 of 21 patients showed rising hCG titers through the third dose of methotrexate. The reported success rate using this regimen was 95%, with a marked reduction in side effects when compared with the series reported by Ory et al (22). The single failure reported was a patient who had fetal cardiac activity in the ectopic pregnancy, with an initial hCG titer of 59,000 mIU/mL. Thus these authors suggested that fetal cardiac activity should be a contraindication to methotrexate initiation.

As experience with a greater number of patients was reported, it seemed that intramuscular methotrexate represented the best route for methotrexate administration in terms of ease of use, incidence of side effects, and success rates. In addition, it appeared that, if the 95% success rate could be upheld, methotrexate would represent an attractive alternative to surgery. Based on these developments, Stovall (7) began a prospective trial in which patients were treated in a similar method to that employed by Sauer et al (24). This protocol differed, however, in that patients were given methotrexate only until their hCG titer began to fall; all patients were treated on an outpatient basis. The initial report suggested that the treatment protocol was both safe and effective and produced only minimal side effects, none of which was hematologic in nature. As a result, the timing and amount of laboratory data collected were adjusted downward to make the protocol more acceptable to patients and to make it more cost-effective.

Table 5.1 describes the revised treatment protocol. If the multidose protocol is followed, citrovorum factor should always be given on the day following methotrexate, even if no further methotrexate is indicated. After discontinuation of methotrexate/citrovorum factor, hCG titers are obtained every seven days until levels fall below 12 mIU/mL. A second

TABLE 5.1

Multidose Protocol for Treatment of Unruptured Ectopic Pregnancy

DAY	TIME	THERAPY
1	Variable	CBC, SGOT, MTX, hCG, blood type + Rh, BUN, creatinine
2	8:00 A.M.	CF, hCG
3	8:00 A.M.	MTX, hCG
4	8:00 A.M.	CF, hCG
5	8:00 A.M.	MTX, hCG
6	8:00 A.M.	CF, hCG
7	8:00 A.M.	MTX, hCG
8	8:00 A.M.	CF, hCG

CBC = complete blood count with differential and platelet count; SGOT = serum glutamic oxalacetic transaminase, units/L; MTX = intramuscular methotrexate, 1.0 mg/kg; hCG = quantitative beta-human chorionic gonadotropin, mIU/mL; CF = intramuscular citrovorum, 0.1 mg/kg; BUN = blood urea nitrogen.
SOURCE: Reprinted with permission from Stovall TG, Ling FW, eds. Extrauterine pregnancy: clinical diagnosis and management. New York: McGraw Hill Publishers, 1993.

course of methotrexate and citrovorum is given if the patient shows a plateau or rise in the hCG titer. As long as the hCG titer continues to decline, however, the patient need not receive any additional methotrexate.

Stovall's group treated 100 patients with this multidose regimen, with 96 (96%) responding successfully. Four patients failed on medical therapy and required salpingectomy because of tubal rupture. The only risk factor that was predictive of failure was the presence of cardiac activity in the adnexa. The other variables studied—such as pretreatment hCG level, serum progesterone levels, or ectopic pregnancy size (all were smaller than 3.5 cm in greatest dimension)—were predictive of methotrexate failure (that is, ectopic pregnancy rupture). On the other hand, four of five (80%) patients with cardiac activity in the ectopic pregnancy were successfully treated, one of whom had an hCG titer of 21,000 mIU/mL. Of those patients who responded well, five (5%) patients experienced minor methotrexate-related side effects, including three cases where the side effects may have been aggravated by the patients' abuse of alcohol. Unlike the previously reported protocol of Ory et al (22), which required all patients to receive four methotrexate/citrovorum doses, only 19 of 96 (19.8%) patients successfully treated required four doses; all of the side effects occurred in members of this subgroup. Interestingly, 17 (17.7%) of those successfully treated required only one dose of methotrexate/citrovorum (25).

Although the multidose treatment regimen lasted no longer than the primary treatment regimen used, several important findings concerning medical therapy emerged from this series of patients:

- Patients with unruptured ectopic pregnancies can be safely managed on an outpatient basis, even in an indigent population that is at risk for poor compliance.
- Seventeen percent of patients responded successfully to only a single dose.
- The incidence of both major and minor side effects was much lower than had previously been reported.
- The treatment failure rate was acceptable and comparable to the persistent trophoblastic growth rate after laparoscopic salpingostomy.

- Cardiac activity in the ectopic pregnancy represents a relative contraindication to systemic methotrexate therapy.

About the time that the treatment of these 100 patients was ending, the authors became aware of the report by Homesley et al (26), which described the treatment of patients with nonmetastatic gestational trophoblastic disease with methotrexate and citrovorum rescue. In this protocol, patients received an increasing dose of methotrexate, beginning at 35 mg/m^2 and escalating weekly by 5 mg/m^2 to a maximum dose of 50 mg/m^2. Patients tolerated the maximum dose well and experienced few side effects.

Single-dose methotrexate for ectopic pregnancy treatment was first reported by Stovall et al (27). The initial report described 31 patients treated with a single injection of 50 mg/m^2 without citrovorum rescue. One patient withdrew from treatment, leaving 30 patients who completed the protocol. Of these women, 29 (96.7%) were successfully treated. No patient experienced a methotrexate-related side effect, and none required a second dose of methotrexate. In addition, no hematologic changes were noted during the treatment period.

Because the results of this initial experience were very positive, more patients were treated with a protocol that was minimally changed to eliminate an hCG titer on day 2 and hematologic testing on day 7 (Table 5.2). The results of this expanded trial, detailing the results of 120 patients, have been reported (28). All patients had a rising hCG titer at the time of treatment initiation, with the mean hCG titer being 3950 ± 1193 mIU/mL. Patients had a mean age of 26.1 ± 6.2 years, a mean gravidity of 3.2 ± 1.6, and a mean parity of 0.97 ± 1.0. Transvaginal ultrasound visualized cardiac activity in 14 (11.7%) patients, with the ectopic mass being visualized in 113 (94.2%). One patient had a twin ectopic gestation demonstrated by transvaginal scanning, with both embryos having cardiac activity; this patient had a pretreatment hCG titer of 21,200 mIU/mL and responded to a single methotrexate dose. Successful treatment was accomplished in 113 of 120 (94.2%) patients, with the mean time to resolution being 35.5 ± 11.8 days. The mean time to cessation of cardiac activity was 7 days, with a range of 4 to 12 days. The hCG titer increased between days 1 and 4 in 103 (85.8%) subjects. Four (3.3%) patients had a rising hCG titer between days 4 and 7 and required a second methotrexate dose

TABLE 5.2

Single-Dose Protocol for Unruptured Ectopic Pregnancy Treatment

DAY	THERAPY
0	hCG, D&C, CBC, SGOT, BUN, creatinine, blood type + Rh
1	MTX, hCG
4	hCG
7	hCG

If a less than 15% decline in hCG titer is observed between days 4 and 7, give a second dose of methotrexate, 50 mg/m^2, on day 7.

If a 15% or more decline in hCG titer occurs between days 4 and 7, follow the patient weekly until hCG falls below 10 mIU/mL.

Note: In those patients not requiring D&C prior to MTX initiation (hCG less than 2000 mIU/mL and no gestational sac on transvaginal ultrasound), days 0 and 1 are combined.

hCG = quantitative beta-human chorionic gonadotropin, mIU/mL; D&C = dilation and curettage; CBC = complete blood count; SGOT = serum glutamic oxalacetic transaminase, units/L; BUN = blood urea nitrogen; MTX = intramuscular methotrexate, 50 mg/m^2.

SOURCE: Reprinted with permission from Stovall TG, Ling FW, eds. Extrauterine pregnancy: clinical diagnosis and management. New York: McGraw Hill Publishers, 1993.

on day 7. No patient required a third dose of methotrexate, and no patient had an hCG level that plateaued after treatment.

Seven (5.8%) patients required surgical intervention because their ectopic pregnancy ruptured. Two of these women had shown cardiac activity in the ectopic pregnancy. Nausea and vomiting developed in one patient on day 4 of treatment. Her husband was ill with viral gastroenteritis, however, which may have contributed to her symptoms. No other side effects were noted.

It is important to warn patients that they may experience an increase in lower abdominal/pelvic pain during the first one to two weeks following treatment initiation. This phenomenon was observed in patients who received the multidose protocol and in 59.2% of patients treated with this single-dose protocol. Patients are given a nonsteroidal anti-inflammatory agent when treatment begins and often receive Tylenol with codeine if the pain becomes worse. If no relief from the pain occurs, a hematocrit and transvaginal ultrasound are obtained to verify that the ectopic pregnancy has not ruptured. A pelvic examination is not performed, as it could potentially rupture the ectopic pregnancy and adds very little helpful information.

Early in this trial, all patients underwent dilation and suction curettage prior to treatment initiation. In all patients, the pregnancy was determined to be nonviable based on a combination of transvaginal ultrasound findings, serial hCG titers, and serum progesterone levels. Because all viable intrauterine pregnancies at the authors' institution can be visualized at an hCG less than 2000 mIU/mL, we no longer perform a suction curettage on patients with a transvaginal ultrasound showing no gestational fluid collection in association with an hCG titer of 2000 mIU/mL or higher (29). The hCG titer above which all normal intrauterine pregnancies can be visualized via transvaginal ultrasound is specific to each institution. Thus the hCG level that determines whether a suction curettage is performed may vary slightly depending upon experience.

Based on the results obtained with these 120 patients, the single-dose protocol appears to be as effective as the multidose regimen. It has several advantages, however: it requires less methotrexate, does not require citrovorum recovery, reduces patient follow-up compared with the multidose protocol, and is less costly. Like multidose methotrexate, it can be safely completed on an outpatient basis. Single-dose methotrexate also virtually eliminates methotrexate-related side effects. Reflecting this fact, patient acceptance for this treatment option will improve. Single-dose methotrexate is therefore our preferred treatment regimen when methotrexate is to be used (28).

The results from this study were later confirmed by Glock and colleagues. Their investigation treated 35 patients with intramuscular methotrexate (50 mg/m^2). Thirty (85.7%) of these patients were successfully treated, whereas 5 patients failed therapy and required laparoscopic surgery. In this series, 12 (34.3%) patients experienced mild side effects that resolved spontaneously (30). Using the same protocol, Gross et al reported a 94.1% success rate in a community hospital setting (31), and Stika et al reported a 78% overall success rate. The reason for this difference is not known (32).

Using a slightly modified protocol and set of inclusion criteria, Henry and Gentry (33) treated 61 patients with intramuscular methotrexate (50 mg/m^2). Sixteen patients received a second injection when two consecutive hCG titers were rising or plateauing. Patients with fetal cardiac activity in the ectopic pregnancy were excluded from the study. Fifty-two (85%) patients were successfully treated as outpatients with methotrexate alone. In this study, the criteria for treatment failure were also defined differently than in the studies carried out by Stovall et al (28).

Single-dose intramuscular methotrexate (50 mg/m^2) has also been shown to be effective for the treatment of a persistent ectopic pregnancy. When Hoppe et al treated 19 consecutive patients with increasing hCG titers after salpingostomy (34), all of the patients responded well, although one patient experienced a probable self-limited intra–abdominal bleeding episode that required a blood transfusion.

Ideally, one would be able to predict which patients would respond to methotrexate treatment before therapy began. If this type of prediction were possible, then only this group of patients would be treated medically. Based on the results of a very small study, Ransom et al have suggested that a serum progesterone of less than 10 mg/mL might be useful for predicting resolution of the tubal pregnancy. On the other hand, patients with a serum progesterone level exceeding 10 mg/mL also respond successfully to methotrexate therapy (35). Stika et al (32) have suggested that the pretreatment hCG level could be used to predict methotrexate response. In their series, women with a pretreatment hCG level of more than 5000 mIU/mL had a greater probability of requiring surgical intervention or multiple doses of methotrexate. Again, it must be emphasized that patients with hCG levels exceeding 5000 can be successfully treated, and a specific hCG level cannot be used to determine the method of treatment.

Thus, to date the only consistent predictor of decreased success with methotrexate therapy has been ectopic mass greater than 3.5 cm or fetal cardiac activity in the ectopic gestation. Nevertheless, patients can be successfully treated even when these factors are present.

INDICATIONS AND COMPLICATIONS

The use of medical therapy is most appropriate when the diagnosis of ectopic pregnancy can be confirmed nonsurgically. At present, the pharmacologic agent that has attracted the most attention is methotrexate, although other agents such as potassium chloride (KCl), hyperosmolar glucose, prostaglandins, and RU-486 have been investigated as well. These agents can be given both systemically (intravenously, intramuscularly, or orally) and locally (direct injection via laparoscopy or ultrasound, or retrograde using salpingography). Based on the available data, systemic methotrexate appears to represent a viable alternative to laparoscopic surgical management of selected patients with ectopic pregnancy.

To maximize the safety of treatment and to eliminate the possibility of treating nonviable intrauterine or early viable intrauterine pregnancy, it is important to adhere to several basic tenets prior to instituting therapy. At present, patients considered candidates for methotrexate treatment include women with the following characteristics:

- A plateaued or rising hCG titer following salpingostomy
- A rising or plateaued hCG titer at least 12 to 24 hours following suction curettage that failed to reveal chorionic villi
- No intrauterine gestational sac or fluid collection on transvaginal ultrasound, in conjunction with an hCG titer of 2000 mIU/mL or higher
- No desire to preserve fertility (for example, women with previous tubal ligation)

In addition, the ectopic pregnancy mass should be 3.5 cm or less in greatest dimension, as demonstrated by transvaginal ultrasound. The clinician must interpret the ultrasound findings with caution, as the majority of unruptured ectopic pregnancies will have fluid in the cul-de-sac.

Cardiac activity in the ectopic pregnancy remains a relative contraindication to medical therapy, as it is associated with a higher failure rate. Patients who have undergone a previous tubal ligation or prior surgery in the effected fallopian tube are not considered good candidates for treatment. Because these patients are at risk for another ectopic pregnancy, it seems more practical to treat their ectopic surgically and remove their fallopian tubes at the same time. In addition, patients with elevated liver enzymes, thrombocytopenia, or decreased white blood cell counts are ineligible for methotrexate therapy. Women who are hemodynamically unstable must be treated surgically; those with significant pain, signs of peritoneal irritation, and fluid in the cul-de-sac on ultrasound should be treated with methotrexate only with caution, even if they are otherwise stable. Finally, patients who are poor follow-up risks or patients who do not wish to be treated medically should not receive methotrexate. Using these inclusion and exclusion criteria, 42% to 45% of women with an ectopic pregnancy represent candidates for methotrexate therapy (28,30).

After receiving methotrexate, women are followed as outpatients as outlined in Table 5.3. Transvaginal ultrasounds are obtained only in those patients who develop abdominal/pelvic pain that fails to be relieved by a mild narcotic. Brown et al (36) performed serial transvaginal ultrasounds on patients after initiation of methotrexate therapy. The findings were not helpful as a routine addition to patient management. In many patients, the ectopic pregnancy mass increased in size and developed a surrounding hematoma, and the amount of cul-de-sac fluid

---

TABLE 5.3

Instructions Given to Patients at the Time That Intramuscular Methotrexate Is Given

---

Tell the patient to refrain from alcohol use, consumption of multivitamins containing folic acid, and sexual intercourse until the hCG titer is negative.

Tell the patient to call her physician if she experiences prolonged or heavy vaginal bleeding.

Tell the patient that she will probably experience an increase in lower abdominal and pelvic pain during the first 10 to 14 days of treatment. Instruct her to call her physician if the pain is prolonged or severe.

Give instructions for use of oral or barrier contraceptives.

Make sure that all of the patient's questions have been answered.

Note that approximately 5% of women do not respond to methotrexate treatment and require surgery.

SOURCE: Reprinted with permission from Stovall TG, Ling FW, eds. Extrauterine pregnancy: clinical diagnosis and management. New York: McGraw Hill Publishers, 1993.

increased. On the other hand, transvaginal ultrasound proved helpful in those patients who developed severe pain, as it reassured both patient and physician that the ectopic pregnancy had not ruptured. The authors do not intervene surgically based on ultrasound findings unless evidence of ectopic pregnancy rupture (a significant decrease in hematocrit or hemodynamic instability in the patient) becomes apparent.

Patients are given either oral or barrier contraceptive methods and asked not to have intercourse until the hCG titer becomes negative. In addition, they are advised not to become pregnant for two months following treatment completion to avoid a potential theoretical risk that methotrexate might affect the developing ovarian follicle. A hysterosalpingogram is performed during the second menstrual cycle. Although this test is not mandatory, its results are important for research purposes and provide information that can be used for patient counseling.

Although several treatment protocols have been developed, it appears prudent from the clinician's standpoint to use the treatment regimen that has proved most successful and for which the most data have been gathered in terms of treatment and follow-up (that is, either the individualized multidose or single-dose intramuscular protocols).

Before initiating methotrexate, the physician should make certain that he or she has taken the following steps:

1. Obtained hCG titer
2. Performed a transvaginal ultrasound within the previous 48 hours
3. Performed endometrial curettage if the hCG titer was less than 2000 mIU/mL
4. Obtained normal liver function (SGOT), normal renal function (BUN, Cr), and a normal CBC (WBC greater than 2000/mL and platelet count of 100,000 or higher)
5. Gave a rhogam if patient was Rh-negative
6. Documented an unruptured ectopic pregnancy of 3.5 cm or less by transvaginal ultrasound (this measurement includes the ectopic sac, if visible, as well as any surrounding hemorrhage or fluid)
7. Obtained informed consent
8. Administered $FeSO_4$, 325 mg PO bid, if the hematocrit is 30% or less
9. Made follow-up appointments on days 4, 6, and 7

Patient Follow-Up

Following institution of intramuscular methotrexate, patients are followed on an outpatient basis as described in Tables 5.1 and 5.2. Any women who report severe or prolonged pain are evaluated by obtaining a hematocrit and transvaginal ultrasound. The ultrasound findings during follow-up have been described by Brown et al. Although not helpful in the majority of patients, transvaginal ultrasound can nevertheless reassure both patient and physician that the ectopic pregnancy has not ruptured. It is important to realize that cul-de-sac fluid is a very common finding and that the amount of fluid may increase if a tubal abortion occurs. In this case, it is usually unnecessary to intervene surgically unless the patient develops a precipitous drop in hematocrit or becomes hemodynamically unstable.

Patients are asked not to become pregnant for at least two months following completion of treatment so that a hysterosalpingogram can be obtained. Although the procedure is not mandatory, its results are important for research purposes and to provide information that can help predict success for future pregnancies. After methotrexate therapy, Stovall (28) found patency of the ipsilateral fallopian tube in 82.6% of patients; Glock (30) noted patency in 79.6%. The potential for pregnancy after medical therapy is similar to that achieved after surgical treatment.

Oral Methotrexate

Higgins and Schwartz (37) were the first to report the use of oral methotrexate in treating persistent trophoblastic tissue following salpingostomy. In their regimen, the patient received 5 mg of methotrexate for five consecutive days; no citrovorum factor was used. A follow-up hysterosalpingogram demonstrated bilateral tubal patency, and the patient had a subsequent viable intrauterine pregnancy. A second case was reported by Pastner and Kenigsberg (38) using a methotrexate-only regimen of 0.4 mg/kg/day for five consecutive days. Bengtsson and colleagues (39) reported a series of 15 patients treated with oral methotrexate; again, these cases involved persistent trophoblastic tissue. The first five patients treated received only methotrexate, whereas the subsequent five patients took a combination of methotrexate and citrovorum. All patients not receiving citrovorum factor experienced side effects, whereas none of the patients treated with both methotrexate and citrovorum developed side effects.

Although it appears that oral methotrexate will successfully treat persistent trophoblastic tissue after salpingostomy, it is probably appropriate at this time to use citrovorum rescue. Also, the clinician must stress the need for patient compliance, because the patient is required to take a medication at a specific time.

Other Agents and Techniques

Salpingocentesis is a technique in which agents such as KCl, methotrexate, prostaglandins, or hyperosmolar glucose are injected into the ectopic pregnancy. This procedure has been accomplished by transvaginal ultrasound guidance, laparoscopy, and transcervical tubal cannulization.

Injection of KCl or Methotrexate by Ultrasound: To date, 203 cases of salpingocentesis using methotrexate have been reported (Table 5.4) (40–50), with 82 (79.6%) women being successfully treated. Potential

TABLE 5.4

Ultrasound-Directed Injection: Methotrexate

Investigator	Number of Patients	Number Successful	Success Rate (%)	Tubal Patency Number	Tubal Patency (%)	Side Effects
Fernandez, 1991 (40)	12	8	76	7	88	1
Menard, 1990 (41)	17	17	100	—	—	0
Feichtinger, 1987 (42)	9	8	89	—	—	0
Leeton, 1988 (43)	2	2	100	—	—	0
Robertson, 1987 (44)	3	1	33	—	—	0
Tulandi, 1991 (45)	12	10	100	—	100	0
Clark, 1989 (46)	1	1	—	1/1	—	0
Porreco, 1992 (47)	3	3	100	0/1	0	0
Timor-Tritsch, 1989 (48)	4	4	100	—	—	0
Tulandi, 1992 (49)	40	28	70	9/11	82	0
Fernandez, 1993 (50)	100	83	83	72/80	90	0
Total	203	165	81.3	89/100	89	1

SOURCE: Reprinted with permission from Stovall TG, Ling FW, eds. Extrauterine pregnancy: clinical diagnosis and management. New York: McGraw Hill Publishers, 1993.

TABLE 5.5

Ultrasound-Directed Injection: Potassium Chloride, Prostaglandin E_2

Drug and Investigator	Number of Patients	Number Successful	Success Rate (%)	Tubal Patency Number	Tubal Patency (%)	Side Effects
KCl						
Timor-Tritsch, 1992 (51)	1	1	100	—	—	0
Binder, 1992 (52)	2	0	0	—	—	0
Oelsner, 1993 (53)	1	1	100	—	—	0
PGE$_2$						
Ribic-Paucel, 1989 (54)	2	0	0	—	—	0
Feichtinger, 1989 (55)	1	0	0	—	—	1
Fernandez, 1991 (40)	9	6	67	6	100	0

SOURCE: Reprinted with permission from Stovall TG, Ling FW, eds. Extrauterine pregnancy: clinical diagnosis and management. New York: McGraw Hill Publishers, 1993.

advantages to this technique include a one-time injection, with the avoidance of potential systemic complications of methotrexate. Reproductive function following this form of treatment has yet to be reported. Because of the limited experience reported so far, this form of treatment cannot be recommended until further studies are completed. Other agents used have included KCl and prostaglandin E_2 (PGE$_2$) (Table 5.5) (40,51–55).

Injection at Laparoscopy: Agents injected into the amniotic sac at laparoscopy have included PGE$_2$, PGF$_{2\alpha}$ (Table 5.6) (56–63), hyperosmolar glucose (see Table 5.6), and methotrexate (Table 5.7) (64–69). This method has the obvious disadvantage of requiring laparoscopy, but can be readily performed if laparoscopy has already been selected. Two cases of cardiac arrhythmia and one case of transitory hypertension, with pulmonary edema and atrioventricular block, have been reported. These effects may be related to extravasation of PGE$_{2\alpha}$ into surrounding blood vessels.

Transcervical Cannulation: Risquez et al (70) reported a multicenter trial in which 31 patients with an ectopic pregnancy were treated using a technique of transcervical cannulation followed by intraluminal methotrexate injection. This technique requires fluoroscopic guidance. The dose of

TABLE 5.6

Laparoscopic Injection: Prostaglandin and Hyperosmolar Glucose

Drug and Investigator	Number of Patients	Number Successful	Success Rate (%)	Tubal Patency Number	Tubal Patency (%)	Side Effects
Local PGF$_{2\alpha}$ and systemic PGE$_2$						
Lindblom, 1987 (56)	26	24	92	—	—	0
Egarter, 1989 (57,58)	71	57	81	22/24	92	3
Vejtorp, 1989 (59)	11	10	91	6/7	85	0
Paulsson, 1995 (60)	127	120	93	—	—	0
Hyperosmolar glucose						
Lang, 1989 (61)	9	9	100	3/3	100	0
Lang, 1992 (62)	60	55	91.7	—	—	0
Yeko, 1995 (63)	16	15	94	10	100	0

SOURCE: Reprinted with permission from Stovall TG, Ling FW, eds. Extrauterine pregnancy: clinical diagnosis and management. New York: McGraw Hill Publishers, 1993.

methotrexate varied from 5 to 50 mg, with the exact amount being left to the discretion of the investigator. Twenty-seven (87%) patients had complete resolution of the ectopic pregnancy. Follow-up was limited to seven patients who had normal hysterosalpingograms and five patients who had an intrauterine pregnancy.

Combined KCl Methotrexate Direct Injection: Guingis (71) reported five cases treated by aspiration of the ectopic gestational sac and injection of KCl and methotrexate. These cases were diagnosed by transvaginal ultrasound. All five cases involved viable ectopic pregnancies with a detectable fetal heartbeat. Four patients did not require any further treatment. In the fifth patient, salpingectomy was performed because of a persistent tubal mass and pain. No systemic side effects were seen.

Abolghar et al (72) reported the successful resolution of an ectopic gestation with a demonstrable fetal heartbeat after injection of 2 mEq/mL KCl and 12.5 mg methotrexate into the amniotic sac. Transvaginal ultrasound was employed both to make the diagnosis of ectopic gestation and to perform the procedure. No chemotherapy-related side effects were noted.

TABLE 5.7

Laparoscopic Injection: Methotrexate

Investigator	Number of Patients	Number Successful	Success Rate (%)	Tubal Patency Number	Tubal Patency (%)	Side Effects
Kijima, 1990 (64)	9	9	100	9/9	100	0
Pansky, 1989 (65)	27	24	88	19/21	90	0
Zakut, 1989 (66)	10	8	80	7/7	100	1
Kooi, 1990 (67)	25	24	96	—	—	5
Mottla, 1992 (68)	7	3	43	—	—	0
Wolf, 1991 (69)	9	8	—	—	—	0
Total	87	76	87.4	35/37	94.6	6

SOURCE: Reprinted with permission from Stovall TG, Ling FW, eds. Extrauterine pregnancy: clinical diagnosis and management. New York: McGraw Hill Publishers, 1993.

Actinomycin D: A single case report has surfaced regarding the use of actinomycin D for primary ectopic pregnancy treatment (73). The patient received four 0.5 mg courses of actinomycin D intravenously daily for five days, with a one-week interval between courses. The patient experienced no serious side effects but did develop nausea.

Actinomycin D represents an alternative agent for treating gestational trophoblastic disease and may be useful for ectopic pregnancy. Only minimal data are available for this application, however. Also, this drug must be given intravenously, and the only report available suggests that prolonged treatment courses will be required.

RU-486: RU-486 is an antiprogesterone that has been used as an abortifacient agent in early intrauterine pregnancies. No cases of primary therapy and only one case of residual ectopic pregnancy have been reported. In this reported case (74), the patient received a single 650-mg oral dose — the same dose used for intrauterine pregnancy termination. One week later, the hCG titers were unchanged. This patient was subsequently treated successfully with methotrexate. It is possible that a second or higher dose might have proved successful. Currently, RU–486 is not available in the United States and cannot be recommended as part of medical therapy.

Anti-hCG Antibody: In an attempt to develop an immunotherapeutic approach to ectopic pregnancy treatment, Frydman et al (75) conducted a Phase 1 clinical trial using mouse monoclonal anti–hCG antibody directed to an antigenic site on the α-subunit of hCG. Three patients with laparoscopically proven ampullary ectopic pregnancies received either a 5-mg or a 25-mg intravenous dose. Only one patient was successfully treated; the other two patients required salpingectomy because of persistent hCG titers. Additional data must be reported before this agent can be incorporated into the treatment regimen for ectopic pregnancy.

PERSISTENT ECTOPIC PREGNANCY

Persistent trophoblastic proliferation following salpingostomy is a well-recognized complication of conservative surgical management, affecting approximately 5% of patients so treated (76). When it occurs, two alternatives are available: 1) reoperation with attempted removal of the trophoblastic tissue or salpingectomy, or 2) medical therapy. A nonsurgical approach would seem preferable, as it has a better chance of preserving reproductive function in this group of women and avoids the problem of reoperation.

Several case reports have been published (39,77–81) regarding various treatment regimens and routes of administration. Dumesic and Hafez (81) reported the only failure of medical therapy after conservative surgery. This patient received methotrexate (1.0 mg/kg intramuscularly), with citrovorum factor (0.1 mg/kg intramuscularly) rescue beginning on the eighth postoperative day. On the eleventh day, the patient became symptomatic and required salpingectomy.

The authors have successfully used a single-dose methotrexate regimen to treat three cases of persistent ectopic pregnancy (28). None of these patients developed methotrexate-related side effects. Like patients treated primarily, however, these women experienced increased lower abdominal discomfort and pain during treatment. Based on the currently available data, methotrexate appears to represent an alternative to surgical retreatment and offers the patient distinct advantages.

COMPARISON TO SURGICAL TREATMENT

No studies published to date have directly compared intramuscular methotrexate and laparoscopic salpingostomy. Instead, all studies have been performed in different patient populations and inclusion criteria for laparoscopic surgery have often varied from the inclusion criteria used for medical treatment. Nevertheless, it appears that intramuscular methotrexate has similar treatment outcomes to surgery. It is certainly a cost-effective treatment model and offers advantages to selected patients with an ectopic pregnancy (82,83). The cost-effectiveness of methotrexate has been confirmed by Alexander et al, who found that the use of methotrexate compared to laparoscopic treatment was associated with a significant cost reduction (84).

In a very limited trial, laparoscopic injection of methotrexate was found to produce results similar to those obtained with laparoscopic linear salpingostomy. Because of the limited number of patients reported, however, no firm conclusions can be drawn (85).

REFERENCES

1. Stovall TG, Ling FW, Carson SA, Buster JE. Nonsurgical diagnosis and treatment of tubal pregnancy. Fertil Steril 1990;54:537.
2. Stovall TG, Ling FW. Ectopic pregnancy: diagnostic and therapeutic algorithms minimizing surgical intervention. J Reprod Med 1993;38:807.
3. Stovall TG, Kellerman AL, Ling FW, Buster JE. Emergency department diagnosis of ectopic pregnancy. Ann Emerg Med 1990;19:1098.
4. Stovall TG, Ling FW, Cope BJ, Buster JE. Preventing ruptured ectopic pregnancy with a single serum progesterone. Am J Obstet Gynecol 1989;160:1435.
5. Stovall TG, Ling FW, Andersen RN, Buster JE. Improved sensitivity and specificity of a single serum progesterone over serial quantitative beta-human chorionic gonadotropin in the screening for ectopic pregnancy. Human Reprod 1992;7:723.

6. Stovall TG, Ling FW, Carson SA, Buster JE. Serum progesterone and uterine curettage in the differential diagnosis of ectopic pregnancy. Fertil Steril 1992;57:456.

7. Stovall TG, Ling FW, Buster JE. Outpatient chemotherapy of unruptured ectopic pregnancy. Fertil Steril 1989;51:435.

8. Li MC, Hertz R, Spencer DB. Effects of methotrexate therapy on choriocarcinoma and chorioadenoma. Proc Soc Biol Med 1956;93:361.

9. Sand PK, Stubblefield PA, Ory SJ. Methotrexate inhibition of normal trophoblasts in vitro. Am J Obstet Gynecol 1986;155:324.

10. Searles G, McKendry RJ. Methotrexate pneumonitis in rheumatoid arthritis: potential risk factors — four case reports and a reviewing of the literature. J Rheumatol 1987;14:1164.

11. Schenfeld A, Mashiach R, Vardy M, Ovadia J. Methotrexate pneumonitis in nonsurgical treatment of ectopic pregnancy. Obstet Gynecol 1992;80:520.

12. Bleyer WA. The clinical pharmacology of methotrexate: New applications of an old drug. Cancer 1978;41:36.

13. Berkowitz RS, Goldstein DP, Jones MA, et al. Methotrexate with citrovorum factor rescue: reduced chemotherapy toxicity in the management of gestational trophoblastic neoplasms. Cancer 1980;45:423.

14. Walden PA, Bagshawe KD. Reproductive performance of women successfully treated for gestational trophoblastic tumors. Am J Obstet Gynecol 1976;125:1108.

15. Van Thiel DH, Ross GT, Lipsett MB. Pregnancies after chemotherapy of trophoblastic neoplasms. Science 1970;169:1326.

16. Rustin GJ, Rustin F, Dent J, et al. No increase in second tumors after cytotoxic chemotherapy for gestational trophoblastic tumors. N Engl J Med 1983;308:473.

17. Tanaka T, Hayaski H, Kutsuzawa T, et al. Treatment of interstitial ectopic pregnancy with methotrexate: report of a successful case. Fertil Steril 1982;37:851.

18. Chotiner JC. Nonsurgical management of ectopic pregnancy associated with severe hyperstimulation syndrome. Obstet Gynecol 1985;66:740.

19. Brandes MC, Youngs DD, Goldstein DP, Parmby TH. Treatment of cornual pregnancy with methotrexate: case report. Am J Obstet Gynecol 1986;1551:655.

20. Haans LCF, Van Kessel PH, Kock HCLV. Treatment of ectopic pregnancy with methotrexate. Eur J Obstet Gynecol Reprod Biol 1987;24:63.

21. Miyazaki Y. Nonsurgical therapy of ectopic pregnancy. Hokkaido Igaku Zasshi 1983;58:132.

22. Ory SJ, Villanueva AL, Sand PK, Tamura RK. Conservative treatment of ectopic pregnancy with methotrexate. Am J Obstet Gynecol 1986;154:1299.

23. Ichinoe K, Wake N, Shinkai N, et al. Nonsurgical therapy to preserve oviduct function in patients with tubal pregnancies. Am J Obstet Gynecol 1987;156:484.

24. Sauer MV, Gorrill MJ, Rodi IA, et al. Nonsurgical management of unruptured ectopic pregnancy: an extended clinical trial. Fertil Steril 1987;48:752.

25. Stovall TG, Ling FW, Gray LA, et al. Methotrexate treatment of unruptured ectopic pregnancy: a report of 100 cases. Obstet Gynecol 1991;77:749.

26. Homesley HD, Blessing JA, Nettenmaier M, Capizzi RL, Major JF, Twiggs LB. Weekly intramuscular methotrexate for nonmetastatic gestational trophoblastic disease. Obstet Gynecol 1988;72:413.

27. Stovall TG, Ling FW, Gray LA. Single-dose methotrexate treatment of ectopic pregnancy. Obstet Gynecol 1991;77:754.

28. Stovall TG, Ling FW. Single dose methotrexate: an expanded clinical trial. Am J Obstet Gynecol 1993;168:1759.

29. Emerson DS, Cartier MS, Altieri LA, et al. Diagnostic efficacy of endovaginal color flow Doppler in an ectopic pregnancy screening program. Radiology 1992;183:413.

30. Glock JL, Johnson JV, Rumsted JR. Efficacy and safety of single-dose systemic methotrexate in the treatment of ectopic pregnancy. Fertil Steril 1994;62:716.

31. Gross Z, Rodriguez JJ, Stalnaker BL. Ectopic pregnancy: nonsurgical, outpatient evaluation and single-dose methotrexate treatment. J Reprod Med 1995;40:371.

32. Stika CS, Anderson L, Frederiksen MC. Single-dose methotrexate for the treatment of ectopic pregnancy: Northwestern Memorial Hospital three-year experience. Am J Obstet Gynecol 1996;174:1840.

33. Henry MA, Gentry WL. Single injection of methotrexate for treatment of ectopic pregnancies. Am J Obstet Gynecol 1994;171:1484.

34. Hoppe DE, Bekkar BE, Nager CW. Single-dose systemic methotrexate for the treatment of persistent ectopic pregnancy after conservative surgery. Obstet Gynecol 1994;83:51.

35. Ransom MX, Garcia AJ, Bohrer M, Corsan GH, Kemman E. Serum progesterone as a predictor of methotrexate success in the treatment of ectopic pregnancy. Obstet Gynecol 1994;83:1033.

36. Brown DL, Felker RE, Stovall TG, et al. Serial endovaginal sonography of ectopic pregnancies treated with methotrexate. Obstet Gynecol 1991;77:406.

37. Higgins KA, Schwartz MB. Treatment of persistent trophoblastic tissue after salpingostomy with methotrexate. Fertil Steril 1986;45:427.
38. Pastner B, Kenigsberg D. Successful treatment of persistent ectopic pregnancy with oral methotrexate. Fertil Steril 1988;6:982.
39. Bengtsson G, Bryman I, Thorburn J, Lindblom B. Low-dose oral methotrexate as second-line therapy for persistent trophoblast after conservative treatment of ectopic pregnancy. Obstet Gynecol 1991;79:589.
40. Fernandez H, Baton C, Lelaidier C, Frydman R. Conservative management of ectopic pregnancy: prospective randomized clinical trial of methotrexate versus prostaglandin sulprostone by combined transvaginal and systemic administration. Fertil Steril 1991;55:746.
41. Menard A, Crequat J, Mandelbrot L, et al. Treatment of unruptured tubal pregnancy by local injection of methotrexate under transvaginal sonographic control. Fertil Steril 1990;54:47.
42. Feichtinger W, Kemeter P. Conservative treatment of ectopic pregnancy by transvaginal aspiration under sonographic control and methotrexate injection. Lancet 1987;1:381.
43. Leeton J, Davison G. Nonsurgical management of unruptured tubal pregnancy with intra-amniotic methotrexate: preliminary report of two cases. Fertil Steril 1988;50:167.
44. Robertson DE, Moye MA, Hansen JH, Serhai P, Swith W, Brinsdew PR, et al. Reduction of ectopic pregnancy by injection under ultrasound control. Lancet 1987;1:974.
45. Tulandi T, Bret PM, Atri M, Senterman M. Treatment of ectopic pregnancy by transvaginal intratubal methotrexate administration. Obstet Gynecol 1991; 77:627.
46. Clark LC, Raymond S, Stranger J, Jackel G. Treatment of ectopic pregnancy with intraamniotic methotrexate: a case report. Aust NZ J Obstet Gynaecol 1989;29:84.
47. Porreco RP. Percutaneous, ultrasound-directed ablation of ectopic pregnancy with methotrexate: a report of three cases. J Reprod Med 1992;37:363.
48. Timor-Tritsch I, Baxi L, Peisner DB. Transvaginal salpingocentesis: a new technique for treating ectopic pregnancy. Am J Obstet Gynecol 1989;160:459.
49. Tulandi T, Atri M, Bret P, et al. Transvaginal intratubal methotrexate treatment of ectopic pregnancy. Fertil Steril 1992;58:98.
50. Fernandez H, Benifla J, Lelaipier C, Baton C, Frydman R. Methotrexate treatment of ectopic pregnancy: 100 cases treated by primary transvaginal injection under sonographic control. Fertil Steril 1993;59:773.

51. Timor-Tritsch IE, Montequdo A, Matera C, Veit CR. Sonographic evolu-
ation of cornual pregnancies treated without surgery. Obstet Gynecol
1992;79:1044.

52. Binder D, Oelsner G, Abmon D, Levran D, Goldenberg M, Mordechai M.
Unsuccessful methotrexate treatment of a tubal pregnancy with a live embryo.
Eur J Obstet Gynecol Reprod Biol 1992;46:154.

53. Oelsner G, Abmon D, Shalev E, Shalev Y, Kukia E, Mashiach S. A new
approach for the treatment of interstitial pregnancy. Fertil Steril 1993;59:707.

54. Ribic-Paucel JM, Novak-Antolic Z, Urhovec I. Treatment of ectopic
pregnancy with prostaglandin E_2. Clin Exp Obstet Gynecol 1989;16:106.

55. Feichtinger W, Kemeter P. Treatment of unruptured ectopic pregnancy by
needling of sac and injection of methotrexate of PGE_2 under transvaginal
sonography control. Arch Gynecol Obstet 1989;246:85.

56. Lindblom B, Kalklfet B, Hahlin M, Hamberger L. Local prostaglandin $F2\alpha$
injection for termination of ectopic pregnancy. Lancet 1987;1:776.

57. Egarter C, Fitz R, Spona J, et al. Treatment of tubal pregnancy with
prostaglandins: a multicenter study. Geburtshilfe Frauenheilkd 1989;49:808.

58. Egarter C, Husslein P. Treatment of tubal pregnancy by prostaglandin.
Lancet 1989;May:276.

59. Vejtorp M, Vejerslev LO, Ruge S. Local prostaglandin treatment of ectopic
pregnancy. Hum Reprod 1989;4:464.

60. Paulsson G, Kvint S, Labecker B, et al. Laparoscopic prostaglandin injection
in ectopic pregnancy: success rates according to endocrine activity. Fertil
Steril 1995;63:473.

61. Lang P, Weiss PAM, Mayer HO. Local application of hyperosmolar glucose
solution in tubal pregnancy. Lancet 1989;2:922.

62. Lang PF, Tamussino K, Honigl W, Ralph G. Treatment of unruptured tubal
pregnancy by laparoscopic instillation of hyperosmolar glucosal solution.
Obstet Gynecol 1992;166:1378.

63. Yeko TR, Mayer JC, Parsons AK, Maroulis GB. A prospective series of
unruptured ectopic pregnancies treated by tubal injection with hyperosmolar
glucose. Obstet Gynecol 1995;85:265.

64. Kijima E, Abe Y, Morita M, et al. The treatment of unruptured tubal
pregnancy with intratubal methotrexate injection under laparoscopic control.
Obstet Gynecol 1990;75:723.

65. Pansky M, Bukovsky I, Golan A, et al. Local methotrexate injection: a nonsurgical treatment of ectopic pregnancy. Am J Obstet Gynecol 1989;161:393.

66. Zakut H, Sadan O, Katz A, et al. Management of tubal pregnancy with
methotrexate. Br J Obstet Gynaecol 1989;96:725.

67. Kooi S, Lock HCLV. Treatment of tubal pregnancy by local injection of methotrexate after adrenaline injection into the mesosalpinx: a report of 25 patients. Fertil Steril 1990;54:580.

68. Mottla GL, Rulin MC, Guzick DS. Lack of resolution of ectopic pregnancy by intratubal injection of methotrexate. Fertil Steril 1992;57:685.

69. Wolf GC, Witt BR. Outpatient laparoscopic management of ectopic pregnancy with a local methotrexate injection. J Reprod Med 1991;36:489.

70. Risquez F, Forman R, Maleiha F, et al. Transcervical cannulation of the fallopian tube for the management of ectopic pregnancy: prospective multicenter study. Fertil Steril 1992;58:1131.

71. Guingis RR. Simultaneous intrauterine and ectopic pregnancies following in-vitro fertilization and gamete intra-fallopian transfer: a review of nine cases. Hum Reprod 1990;5:484.

72. Abolghar MA, Mansour RT, Serour GI. Transvaginal injection of potassium chloride and methotrexate for the treatment of tubal pregnancy with a live fetus. Hum Reprod 1990;5:887.

73. Altarus M, Cohen I, Corduba M, et al. Treatment of an interstitial pregnancy with actinomycin D. Case report. Br J Obstet Gynaecol 1988;95:1321.

74. Kenigsberg D, Porte J, Hull M, Spitz IM. Medical treatment of residual ectopic pregnancy: RU 486 and methotrexate. Fertil Steril 1987;47:702.

75. Frydman R, Fernandez H, Troalen F, et al. Phase I clinical trial of monoclonal antihuman chorionic gonadotropin antibody in women with an ectopic pregnancy. Fertil Steril 1989;52:734.

76. Vermesh M. Conservative management of ectopic gestation. Fertil Steril 1989;51:550.

77. Hill GA, Cartwright PS, Herbert CM. Retained trophoblast conservative management of ectopic pregnancy: a report of two cases. J Reprod Med 1990;35:415.

78. Rose PG, Cohen SM. Methotrexate therapy for persistent ectopic pregnancy after conservative laparoscopic surgery. Obstet Gynecol 1990;76:947.

79. Cowan BD, McGehee RP, Bates GW. Treatment of persistent ectopic pregnancy with methotrexate and leukovorum rescue: a case report. Obstet Gynecol 1986;67:50S.

80. DiMarchi JM, Cyka RE. Oral methotrexate for persistent ectopic pregnancy: a case. J Reprod Med 1992;37:659.

81. Dumesic DA, Hafez GR. Delayed hemorrhage of a persistent ectopic pregnancy following laparoscopic salpingostomy and methotrexate therapy. Obstet Gynecol 1991;78:960.

82. Creinin MD, Washington AE. Cost of ectopic pregnancy management: surgery versus methotrexate. Fertil Steril 1993;60:963.

83. Stovall TG, Bradham DD, Ling FW, Naughton M. Cost of treatment of ectopic pregnancy: single-dose methotrexate versus surgical treatment. J Women's Health 1994;3:445.

84. Alexander JM, Rouse DJ, Varner E, Austin JM. Treatment of the small unruptured ectopic pregnancy. A cost analysis of methotrexate versus laparoscopy. Obstet Gynecol 1996;88:123.

85. Porpora MG, Oliva M, Decatstofar A, et al. Comparison of local injection of methotrexate and linear salpingostomy in the conservative laparoscopic treatment of ectopic pregnancy. J Am Assoc Gyn Lapar 1996;3:271.

6

Salpingocentesis

Togas Tulandi

T he traditional treatment of ectopic pregnancy (EP) involves laparotomy and removal of the affected tube. Advances in ultrasound technology, however, enable EP to be detected much earlier, which has allowed conservative treatment without removing the tube. Preserving the tube increases the chance of subsequent live births. In addition, more conservative treatment approaches have been advocated, including expectant and medical management. Medical treatment can be given systemically or locally into the ectopic gestation. Local treatment decreases systemic side effects and leads to a higher concentration of drugs locally. With this approach, the objectives are complete destruction of the trophoblastic tissue and maximal preservation of the reproductive function in the affected tube.

METHOTREXATE

Local Treatment with Methotrexate

One of the most widely used drugs for local treatment of EP is methotrexate (MTX). MTX is a folic acid reductase inhibitor that induces dissolution of trophoblastic tissue. It can be administered by laparoscopy, transvaginally under ultrasound guidance, or transcervically under fluoroscopic or ultrasound control.

Laparoscopic Intratubal MTX

Several investigators have reported encouraging results of treatment of EP by local injection of MTX at laparoscopy (1–4). Under laparoscopic control, MTX (12.5–25.0 mg) is simply injected into the tubal pregnancy. Pansky et al (2) reported an intrauterine pregnancy rate after treatment of 67% and a recurrent ectopic pregnancy rate of 13%. Mottla et al (5) conducted a randomized trial comparing the efficacy of laparoscopic removal of EP and laparoscopic intratubal MTX. The group terminated its study prematurely because of the disappointing results in the MTX group. Of seven patients, three required another surgery and another had persistent EP requiring systemic MTX administration. When another randomized study compared the effects of laparoscopic intratubal injection of MTX and salpingotomy (3), the results were similar. The authors stated that laparoscopic salpingotomy or salpingectomy can be used in most cases, whereas MTX has a more selective application. They restricted their use of this drug to unruptured tubal pregnancy of less than 4 cm in diameter.

Shalev et al (4) treated 44 women with local injection of methotrexate at laparoscopy and 55 women with salpingotomy. The investigators found that treatment was successful in 27 of 44 women (61.4%) in the methotrexate group and in 51 of 55 (92.7%) in the salpingotomy group. The failure rate fell from 48.1% to 23.5% if the tubal diameter was limited to less than 2 cm and from 71.4% to 23.3% if the serum β-hCG levels were less than 2000 mIU/mL. No significant difference was noted in the tubal patency rate, intrauterine pregnancy rate, or recurrent ectopic pregnancy rate between the methotrexate group and the salpingotomy group. The results of this study suggest that local methotrexate administration is effective and safe in a selected group of patients. Nevertheless, this method of treatment still requires a laparoscopy.

When Shulman et al (6) studied the effects of MTX on corpus luteum activity, they failed to find any correlation between the success of treatment and the pattern of serum estradiol, progesterone, and β-hCG levels. Three of seven patients who received local MTX and two of eight patients who received both local and systemic MTX experienced an initial rise in β-hCG levels. In these women, increasing levels of the three hormones were seen in patients who received local therapy, but decreases in estradiol and progesterone levels were encountered in those who also received systemic treatment. The researchers postulated that systemic — but not local — MTX administration might have some effect on the corpus luteum activity.

Local treatment of EP by laparoscopy is simple and does not require a higher degree of technical skills and a greater variety of equipment than does diagnostic laparoscopy or tubal sterilization. Nevertheless, this approach requires a laparoscopy and general anesthesia. Furthermore, its use is limited to a selected group of patients with EP.

Transvaginal Intratubal MTX

Local transvaginal MTX treatment represents an attractive alternative to laparoscopic administration of methotrexate. It does not require surgery and general anesthesia. Mènard et al (7) found that resolution of tubal pregnancy occurred in 13 of 17 patients who were treated by transvaginal MTX under ultrasound guidance. The study did not measure serum β-hCG levels before the treatment began. Tulandi et al (8) found that transvaginal MTX treatment of EP in 40 women who had increasing serum β-hCG levels was associated with a high failure rate (30%). Furthermore, the affected tubes became distended before gradually decreasing in size, and they remained distended long after the serum β-hCG became undetectable.

Fernandez et al (9) used a scoring system involving six parameters graded on a scale from 1 to 3: gestational age, serum β-hCG level, serum progesterone level, abdominal pain, hemoperitoneum, and tubal diameter. They found that the success rate of local transvaginal MTX treatment (1 mg/kg body weight) was 90% when the patient's score was 13 or less. Subsequently, these researchers conducted a randomized study comparing this treatment with laparoscopic salpingotomy in women with a score of 13 or less (10). The two treatments were equally successful. As expected, the serum β-hCG levels returned to undetectable levels faster in the salpingotomy group (methotrexate group, 28.8 days; salpingotomy, 13.6 days).

Interstitial pregnancy has also been successfully treated by local injection of methotrexate (11−13).

It appears that local treatment of EP with methotrexate either by laparoscopy or transvaginally can be effective in a select group of patients.

Because transvaginal treatment is less invasive, it is a better alternative than local laparoscopic treatment.

Transcervical Intratubal MTX

Risquez et al (14) administered MTX (5–50 mg) by transcervical tubal cannulation into the ectopic gestational site under fluoroscopic or ultrasound control. Resolution occurred in 27 of 31 patients (87%). Following the publication of these results, the researchers restricted the treatment to cases where "laparoscopic surgery is difficult to carry out, such as frozen pelvis, angular pregnancy or interstitial pregnancy" (15). In any event, the transvaginal technique is simpler.

PROSTAGLANDIN

Laparoscopic Intratubal Prostaglandin

Local prostaglandin injection by laparoscopy has been reported by several authors (16). The procedure has proved successful in most patients. For example, Egarter et al (17) treated 75 patients with local $PGF_{2\alpha}$ (5–10 mg) and systemic PGE_2 derivative (50 μg). They achieved successful treatment in 84% of patients with serum β-hCG levels of less than 2500 mIU/mL, although the success rate dropped to 25% if the initial levels were higher than 2500 mIU/mL. A combination treatment with higher dose of prostaglandin (local $PGF_{2\alpha}$ of 10–13 mg) and PGE_2 derivative (500 μg) has produced serious cardio-pulmonary side effects, including pulmonary edema.

Spitzer et al (18) treated 33 women with local prostaglandin injection at laparoscopy, finding an overall success rate of 73%. The results were better in those women with declining serum β-hCG before the treatment.

Paulsson et al (19) treated ectopic pregnancy by injecting both the tubal pregnancy and the corpus luteum with $PGF_{2\alpha}$ (1 mg and 0.5 mg, respectively). The investigators suggested that $PGF_{2\alpha}$ administration into the corpus luteum facilitates corpus luteum regression. They reported that the success rate is "acceptable" in women with pretreated serum β-hCG levels of less than 1000 mIU/mL. A success rate of 86.7% (52 of 60 patients) was also reported by Hagstrom et al (20). Of interest, injection of prostaglandin into the corpus luteum has little effect on the function of the corpus luteum (21).

Prostaglandin treatment appears to give results similar to those achieved with local methotrexate. In contrast, local treatment by laparoscopy either with MTX, prostaglandin, or other substances does not appear to be as effective as laparoscopic salpingostomy.

HYPEROSMOLAR GLUCOSE

Laparoscopic Intratubal Hyperosmolar Glucose

Treatment of ectopic pregnancy by laparoscopic intratubal instillation of 50% glucose solution has been reported. Hyperosmolar glucose probably acts by dehydrating the cells and causing necrobiosis of the trophoblastic tissue. In a randomized study of 40 patients, intratubal glucose administration did not show any advantage over salpingostomy (22). The incidence of persistent ectopic pregnancy was 20% in the glucose group and 10% in the salpingostomy group.

Lang et al (23) treated 60 patients with local instillation of glucose by laparoscopy. They found that 49 of 50 patients (90%) with serum β-hCG levels of 2500 mIU/mL or less did not require further treatment. The success rate decreased to 60%, however, if the serum β-hCG levels exceeded 2500 mIU/mL.

Yeko et al (24) reported laparoscopic injection of hyperosmolar glucose in 15 women with serum β-hCG levels of less than 2500 mIU/mL. With the exception of one patient, all of the subjects responded well to the treatment, and the subsequent hysterosalpingography revealed patent tubes. The investigators found two patterns of serum β-hCG levels after the treatment. An immediate fall in β-hCG levels (type I) was encountered in 13 patients, and an initial rise in the levels (type II) occurred in 3 patients. It was postulated that this initial rise occurred because of the release of hormones into the circulation after trophoblastic cell death. Because the patterns of serum β-hCG levels prior to the treatment were not obtained in all patients, this hypothesis may be erroneous. Perhaps

TABLE 6.1

Treatment of Ectopic Pregnancy by Local Administration of Methotrexate, Hyperosmolar Glucose or Prostaglandin

	Number of Subjects	"Resolution"	Tubal Patency	Recurrent Ectopic*
Methotrexate				
Transvaginal				
Tulandi et al (8)	40	28/40 (70%)	9/11 (81.8%)	2/4 (50%)
Fernandez et al (9)	72[a]	72/80 (90%)	65/72 (90.2%)	1/34 (2.9%)
	28[b]	18/28 (64.3%)		
Fernandez et al (10)	20	19/20 (95%)	15/17 (88%)	0
Laparoscopy				
Pansky et al (2)	77	42/58 (72.4%)	39/41 (95%)	6/30 (20%)
O'Shea et al (3)	29	26/29 (89.7%)	14/18 (77.8%)	NA
Shalev et al (4)	44	27/44 (61.4%)	13/19 (68.4%)	2/15 (13.3%)
Glucose				
Yeko et al (24)	16	15/16 (93.7%)	10/10 (100%)	2/5 (40%)
Lang et al (23)	50[c]	49/50 (98%)	18/22 (81.8%)	1/14 (7.1%)
	10[d]	6/10 (60%)		
Laatikainen et al (22)	20	16/20 (80%)	9/13 (69%)	0/4 (0%)
Prostaglandin by laparoscopy				
Paulsson et al (19)	93	77/93 (82.8%)	NA	NA
Vejtorp et al (21)	30	25/30 (83.3%)	12/14 (85.7%)	NA

*Recurrent on the ipsilateral site.

[a]Serum β-hCG < 5000 mIU/mL.

[b]β-hCG > 5000 mIU/mL.

[c]Serum β-hCG < 2500 mIU/mL.

[d]β-hCG > 2500 mIU/mL.

some patients with increasing serum β-hCG levels did not respond immediately to the treatment and the levels continued to rise (type II), whereas patients with declining serum β-hCG levels before treatment continued to show decrease in the hormone levels. Table 6.1 gives the results of local treatment of ectopic pregnancy by methotrexate, prostaglandin, or hyperosmolar glucose.

OTHER SUBSTANCES

Injection of potassium chloride (KCl) into the gestational sac has been employed for selective termination of multifetal pregnancy. It has also been used for local treatment of tubal EP (8,25,26). KCl causes fetal demise, but its mechanism of action in this indication remains unclear. This agent has also been used locally to treat interstitial pregnancy under ultrasound guidance (25,27).

RU-486, a progesterone receptor blocker, has been tried unsuccessfully to treat patients with EP. Its failure may be due to the absence of progesterone receptor expression in the fallopian tubes containing EP (28,29).

Ali (30) reported treatment of tubal pregnancy with local Danazol administration (400 mg). The treatment was successful in all 15 patients, and tubal patency could be demonstrated in 14 of 15 affected tubes. A confirmation of these results by others is still needed, however.

Other substances that have been used locally to treat a tubal pregnancy include actinomycin (31), trichosantin (32), etoposide (33), and 5-fluorouracil (34).

HISTOPATHOLOGIC EXAMINATION OF THE TUBE AFTER LOCAL TREATMENT

A paucity of information exists regarding the integrity of the tube after medical treatment. In rabbits, local injection of methotrexate does not cause either tubal epithelial impairment or adverse effects on fertility (35). Klinkert et al (36) reported on the changes in the tube six months after local MTX administration (5 mg). They found destruction of the tubal mucosa and extensive fibrosis of muscularis and calcification; sclerotic chorionic villi also appeared in the necrotic and fibrotic tubal wall. Kooi et al (37), on the other hand, found complete repair of two fallopian tubes one year after local MTX treatment. Honigl et al (38) reported no persistent damage of the tubal mucosa after local injection of hyperosmolar glucose.

COMPARISON OF LOCAL AND SURGICAL TREATMENT

Table 6.2 indicates the reproductive outcome after systemic treatment with methotrexate, treatment with local methotrexate, and laparoscopic salpingostomy. Note that methotrexate treatment was administered to a selected group of patients, whereas most patients with ectopic pregnancy received laparoscopic treatment. It appears that local methotrexate treatment of ectopic pregnancy is associated with lower pregnancy rates than systemic or surgical treatment. In the presence of persistent bleeding or ruptured tube, a salpingectomy represents a viable alternative. It is also the preferred procedure for women who do not wish to preserve their fertility.

Surgery remains the definitive and universal treatment for ectopic pregnancy, and it can be safely done by laparoscopy. The incidence of persistently elevated serum β-hCG levels in laparoscopy is similar to that observed with laparotomy (5%) and can be treated with a single methotrexate injection.

EXPECTANT MANAGEMENT

A review of the treatment of ectopic pregnancy would not be complete without discussing expectant management. In some cases, EP will resolve spontaneously. It is very likely that recent advances in diagnosing early and unruptured EP have eliminated cases that would have resolved spontaneously.

TABLE 6.2

Reproductive Outcome After Medical Treatment of Ectopic Pregnancy with Systemic and Local Methotrexate and After Laparoscopic Salpingostomy

Treatment	Authors	Total Number of Patients	Number of Patients Attempted Pregnancy	Total Pregnancy	Intrauterine Pregnancy	Ectopic Pregnancy
Systemic methotrexate	Stovall et al (39)	120	49	39/49 (79.6%)	34/49 (69.4%)	5/39 (12.8%)
Local methotrexate	Fernandez et al (9)	100	58	30/58 (51.8%)	27/58 (46.6%)	3/34 (8.8%)
Salpingostomy	Pouly et al (40)	223	118	102/118 (86.4%)	76/118 (64.4%)	26/76 (25.5%)

Methotrexate treatment was administered to a selected group of patients with an ectopic pregnancy that was 3.5 cm or less in greatest diameter. Salpingostomy was performed in most patients with ectopic pregnancy.

In the past few years, several investigators have evaluated the feasibility and safety of expectant treatment of EP. Ylöstalo et al (41) found that 57 of 83 patients (69%) with EP of less than 4 cm in diameter and with declining serum β-hCG levels did not require further intervention. Twenty patients required surgery because of clinical symptoms or rising serum β-hCG levels. One patient had tubal rupture. In a smaller study (42), spontaneous resolution occurred in 27 of 33 women with EP whose serum β-hCG was 2500 mIU/mL or less and declining.

CONCLUSIONS

In evaluating the efficacy of medical treatment of ectopic pregnancy, it is important to note that spontaneous resolution of ectopic pregnancy occurs in most patients with declining serum β-hCG levels. These patients certainly do not require either medical or surgical treatment. Unfortunately, in most publications, the patterns of serum β-hCG levels before treatment are either not available or not reported. Favorable results are achieved in those patients with serum β-hCG levels of 2500 mIU/mL or less.

When laparoscopy reveals an ectopic pregnancy, removal of the ectopic gestation remains the best method of treatment. Because of the simplicity of injecting MTX at laparoscopy, this procedure can be performed by physicians who are not familiar with salpingostomy by laparoscopy. Local injection by laparoscopy appears to preserve the integrity of the tube, but does not offer any clear advantage over salpingostomy (Fig. 6.1).

Alternatively, the physician can attempt local injection under ultrasound guidance. This procedure is less invasive than the laparoscopic approach. A single intramuscular injection of MTX is certainly less time-consuming and less complicated than intratubal injection under ultrasound guidance. More importantly, it gives similar results.

As more evidence is accumulated, it becomes clear that tubal rupture and hemoperitoneum can still occur after expectant or medical management of ectopic pregnancy (43). These treatments should be delivered with utmost care and patients should be closely monitored. Surgical treatment is required when clinically indicated or when the serum β-hCG levels fail to decline and/or the dilated tube in the region of ectopic pregnancy fails to subside.

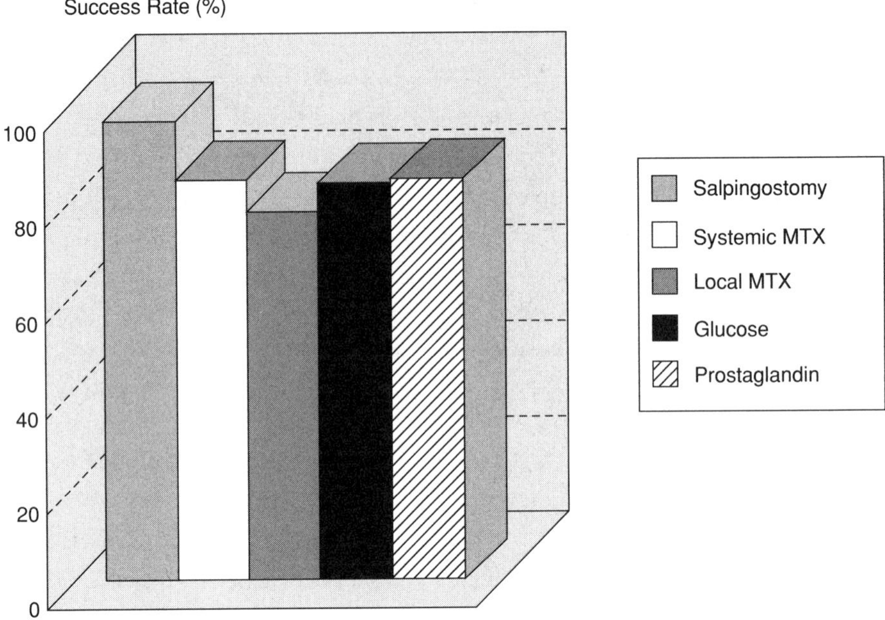

FIG. **6.1.**

"Success rate" after treatment of ectopic pregnancy with laparoscopic salpingostomy, systemic methotrexate, local methotrexate, hyperosmolar glucose, and prostaglandin. Note that the medical treatment was administered to a selected group of patients with an ectopic pregnancy, whereas surgical treatment was performed in most patients with ectopic pregnancy.

REFERENCES

1. Kojima E, Abbe Y, Morita M, Ito M, Hirakawa S, Momose K. The treatment of unruptured tubal pregnancy with intratubal methotrexate injection under laparoscopic control. Obstet Gynecol 1990;75:723.
2. Pansky M, Bukovsky J, Golan A, Avrech O, Langer R, Weinraub Z, Caspi E. Reproductive outcome after laparoscopic local methotrexate injection for tubal pregnancy. Fertil Steril 1993;60:85–87.
3. O'Shea RT, Thompson GR, Harding A. Intra-amniotic methotrexate versus CO_2 laser laparoscopic salpingotomy in the management of tubal ectopic pregnancy—a prospective randomized trial. Fertil Steril 1994;62:876–878.

4. Shalev E, Peleg D, Bustan M, Romano S, Tsabari A. Limited role of intratubal methotrexate treatment of ectopic pregnancy. Fertil Steril 1995;63:20–24.

5. Mottla GL, Rulin MC, Guzick DS. Lack of resolution of ectopic pregnancy by intratubal injection of methotrexate. Fertil Steril 1992;57:685–687.

6. Shulman A, Maymon R, Zmira N, Lotan M, Holtzinger M, Bahary C. Conservative treatment of ectopic pregnancy and its effects on corpus luteum activity. Gynecol Obstet Invest 1992;33:161–164.

7. Mènard A, Crèquat J, Mandelbrot L, Hauuy JP, Medelenat P. Treatment of unruptured tubal pregnancy by local injection of methotrexate under transvaginal sonographic control. Fertil Steril 1990;54:47–50.

8. Tulandi T, Bret P, Atri M, Falcone T, Khalife S. Transvaginal intratubal methotrexate treatment of ectopic pregnancy. Fertil Steril 1992;58:98–100.

9. Fernandez H, Benifla JL, Lelaidier C, Baton C, Frydman R. Methotrexate treatment of ectopic pregnancy: 100 cases treated by primary transvaginal injection under sonographic control. Fertil Steril 1993;59:773–777.

10. Fernandez H, Pauthier S, Doumerc S, Lelaidier C, Olivennes F, Ville Y, Frydman R. Ultrasound guided injection of methotrexate versus laparoscopic salpingotomy in ectopic pregnancy. Fertil Steril 1995;63:25–29.

11. Tanaka T, Hayashi H, Kutsuzawa T, Fujimoto S, Ichinoe K. Treatment of interstitial ectopic pregnancy with methotrexate: report of a successful case. Fertil Steril 1982;37:851.

12. Benifla JL, Sebban E, Pennehouat G, Proust A, Naouri M, Crequat J, Madelenat P. Traitement par le methotrexate de quatre grosesses interstitielles non rompues. Contraception Fertilite Sexualite 1993;21:845–847.

13. Karsdorp VH, Van der Veen F, Schats R, Boer-Meisel ME, Kenemans P. Successful treatment with methotrexate of vital interstitial pregnancy. Human Reprod 1992;7:1164–1169.

14. Risquez F, Forman R, Maleika F, Foulot H, Reidy J, Chapman M, Zorn JR. Transcervical cannulation of the fallopian tube for the management of ectopic pregnancy: prospective multicenter study. Fertil Steril 1992;58:1131–1135.

15. Zorn JR. Dealing with uncertainty — the challenge of the decade? (letter) Fertil Steril 1993;60:1109.

16. Lindblom B, Hahlin M, Lundorff P, Thorburn J. Treatment of tubal pregnancy by laparoscope-guided injection of prostaglandin $F_{2\alpha}$. Fertil Steril 1990;54:404.

17. Egarter C, Kiss H, Vavra N, Husslein P. Reproductive performance after local and systemic prostaglandin for ectopic pregnancy. Arch Gynecol Obstet 1992;252:45–48.

18. Spitzer D, Steiner H, Batka M, Staudach A. Wirksamkeit lokaler prostaglandin—instillationen bei tubargraviditarten in abhangigkeit vom praoperativen beta-hCG verlauf. Zeitschrift für Geburtshilfe und Perinatologie 1992;196:244–246.

19. Paulsson G, Kvint S, Labecker BM, Löfstrand T, Lindblom B. Laparoscopic prostaglandin injection in ectopic pregnancy: success rates according to endocrine activity. Fertil Steril 1995;63:473–477.

20. Hagstrom HG, Hahlin M, Sjoblom P, Lindblom B. Prediction of persistent trophoblastic activity after local prostaglandin F2 alpha injection for ectopic pregnancy. Human Reprod 1994;9:1170–1174.

21. Vejtorp M, Vejerslev LO, Ruge S. Treatment of tubal pregnancy by local injection of prostaglandin: selection of patients and evaluation of subsequent tubal patency. Eur J Obstet Gynecol Reprod Biol 1991;41:85–90.

22. Laatikainen T, Tuomivaara L, Käär K. Comparison of a local injection of hyperosmolar glucose solution with salpingostomy for the conservative treatment of tubal pregnancy. Fertil Steril 1993;60:80–84.

23. Lang PF, Tamussino K, Hönigl W, George R. Treatment of unruptured tubal pregnancy by laparoscopic instillation of hyperosmolar glucose solution. Am J Obstet Gynecol 1992;166:1378–1381.

24. Yeko TR, Mayer JC, Parsons AK, Maroulis GB. Prospective series of unruptured ectopic pregnancies treated by tubal injection with hyperosmolar glucose. Obstet Gynecol 1995;85:265–268.

25. Robertson DE, Smith W, Craft I. Reduction of ectopic pregnancy by injection under ultrasound control. Lancet 1987;1:974.

26. Timor-Tritsch I, Baxi L, Peisner DB. Transvaginal salpingocentesis: a new technique for treating ectopic pregnancy. Am J Obstet Gynecol 1989;160:459.

27. Oelsner G, Admon D, Shalev E, Shalev Y, Kukia E, Mashiach S. A new approach for the treatment of interstitial pregnancy. Fertil Steril 1993;59:924–925.

28. Kenigsberg D, Porte J, Hull M, Spitz IM. Medical treatment of residual ectopic pregnancy: RU 486 and methotrexate. Fertil Steril 1987;47:702.

29. Levin JH, Lacarra M, d'Arblaing G, Grimes DA, Vermesh M. Mefisterone (RU 486) failure in an ovarian heterotopic pregnancy. Am J Obstet Gynecol 1990;163:543.

30. Ali AF. Local Danazol injection for treatment of unruptured tubal pregnancy (preliminary experience). Eur J Obstet Gynecol Reprod Biol 1993;49:137–141.

31. Kooi S, Kock HCLV. A review of the literature on nonsurgical treatment in tubal pregnancies. Obstet Gynecol Survey 1992;47:739–749.

32. Egarter C, Husslein P, Yeung HW. Trichosantin injection in tubal pregnancy. Gynecol Obstet Invest 1991;31:119–120.

33. Kusaka M, Tanaka T, Fujimoto S. Local etoposide injection for the treatment of tubal pregnancy with cardiac activity. Int J Fertil 1994;39:11–13.

34. Xie QH, Liu XC, Liu SY. Injection of 5-fluorouracil in the treatment of tubal pregnancy through salpingo-catheter under hysteroscopy (Chinese). Chinese J Obstet Gynecol 1994;29:106–108.

35. Lecuru F, Buchet-Bouverne B, Querleu D, Bethouart M, Crepin G, Vasquez G. Etude histologique experimentale de la toxicite locale de l'injection intratubaire de methotrexate. J Gynecol Obstet Biol Reprod 1992;21:53–58.

36. Klinkert J, van Geldorp HJ, Chadwa-Ajwani S, Huikeshoven FJM. Tubal damage after intratubal methotrexate treatment. Fertil Steril 1993;59:926–927.

37. Kooi S, van Etten FHPM, Kock HCLV. Histopathology of five tubes after treatment with methotrexate for a tubal pregnancy. Fertil Steril 1992;57:341–345.

38. Honigl W, Pickel H, Tamussino K, Lang PF. Histopathology of the fallopian tube after local instillation of hyperosmolar glucose solution for unruptured tubal pregnancy. Fertil Steril 1993;59:1316–1318.

39. Stovall TG, Ling FW, Gray LA, Carson SA, Buster JE. Methotrexate treatment of unruptured ectopic pregnancy: a report of 100 cases. Obstet Gynecol 1991;77:749–753.

40. Pouly JL, Mahnes H, Mage G, Canis M, Bruhat MA. Conservative laparoscopic treatment of 321 ectopic pregnancies. Fertil Steril 1986;46:1093–1097.

41. Ylöstalo P, Cacciatore B, Sjöberg J, Kääriäinen M, Tenhunen A, Stenman U. Expectant management of ectopic pregnancy. Obstet Gynecol 1992;80:345–348.

42. Makinen JI, Kivijarvi AK, Ifjala KM. Success on non-surgical management of ectopic pregnancy. Lancet 1990;335:1099.

43. Tulandi T, Hemmings R, Khalifa F. Rupture of ectopic pregnancy in women with low and declining serum β-hCG levels. Fertil Steril 1991;56:786–787.

7

Minimally Invasive Extirpative Surgery for Ectopic Pregnancies

Michael P. Diamond

Management of ectopic pregnancies has evolved rapidly over the past two decades. In the early 1970s, the eccyesis was treated at laparotomy, with therapy frequently involving removal of not only the involved fallopian tube, but also the adjacent ovary. Today, in contrast, surgical treatment of tubal ectopic pregnancies rarely includes oophorectomy, frequently is performed endoscopically, and very often involves salpingostomy rather than salpingectomy, particularly in women who desire the capacity for further childbearing. Furthermore, some physicians now advocate alternatives to surgical therapy, such as medical management or even expectant observation, often without surgical diagnostic confirmation of the presence of the eccyesis (the appropriate role for these options remains to be established, however). This chapter will address the role of endoscopic extirpative management of ectopic pregnancies.

Extirpative treatment of ectopic pregnancies can be performed following surgical entry into the abdomen by laparotomy or laparoscopy. The choice of these two options will be based on a variety of factors, including those listed in Table 7.1. Although a number of relative indications exist for treatment by laparotomy, increasingly surgeons are choosing an endoscopic approach. It must be emphasized, however, that no absolute indications have been established for one approach or the other. For most surgeons, a patient with uncontrolled hemorrhage and

TABLE 7.1

Indications for Laparotomy for Treatment of Ectopic Pregnancies

Uncontrolled hemorrhage/hemodynamic shock

Surgeon inexperience with operative laparoscopy

Lack of availability of equipment and instrumentation for performance of operative endoscopy

Lack of availability of experienced nursing personnel/surgical assistants

Pelvic anatomy distortion, including pelvic adhesions

Large ectopic pregnancy

Intraoperative laparoscopic complications or difficulties

hemodynamic instability is a candidate for laparotomy, with the goal being to establish vascular control as quickly as possible. In a limited number of situations involving a very experienced endoscopic surgeon and immediate availability of endoscopic instruments, equipment, and trained assistants, some surgeons would advocate a laparoscopic approach as the quickest way of establishing hemostasis.

A major issue in the decision to perform a laparotomy for ectopic pregnancy should be the experience and expertise of the surgeon, and the available personnel. Unfortunately, some clinicians feel a pressure to perform procedures endoscopically, which they may not be totally qualified to undertake. This pressure, in part, comes from presentations of techniques and videos at national meetings and postgraduate courses by experts in these techniques. Many practitioners will not possess the same expertise and level of experience of these experts, and thus it may be unreasonable for them to set such high expectations for themselves. This decision must be made by each physician and will be likely to vary over time, as the practitioner develops more experience and expertise.

Equally important, but often overlooked, is the experience of the operating room staff. Some hospitals have dedicated nurses for endoscopic surgical procedures. These individuals are often very familiar with the functioning of the high-tech instrumentation used for operative laparoscopy, as well as logistical issues such as the storage location of instruments and devices used during these surgical procedures. When these individuals are not available, as might more frequently occur in evenings, nights, and weekends, the ability to conduct operative laparoscopy may be greatly diminished. Over time, as the progression of endoscopic procedures in other specialties continues to expand an increasing number of operating room nurses will become familiar with the need for operative endoscopy, minimizing this problem. In the meantime, this shortcoming can be addressed in many ways, including having staff on call for endoscopic surgical procedures, scheduling staff so that at least one person who has a knowledge of endoscopic surgery is always available, training all operating personnel, and modifying the mode of entry into the abdomen based on the availability of such personnel. It must be emphasized that having experienced nursing personnel on hand is no substitute for having a surgeon who is familiar with the equipment and instrumentation that will be utilized during the surgical procedure.

One final logistical concern with regard to the choice of mode of entry into the abdominal cavity centers on the available equipment and instrumentation. If their availability is limited in the hospital, and frequently utilized instrumentation or equipment are being used by other physicians or are unavailable because of the need for repair, the need may arise to convert to a laparotomy to perform the surgical procedure.

Ectopic pregnancies frequently occur in women with tubo-peritoneal disease, including prior tubal damage (1). As a result, one may find distortion of the normal pelvic anatomy above and beyond that causing the eccyesis. Consequently, it may be necessary to lyse adhesions to the tube or organs overlying the tube so as to gain access to the ectopic pregnancy. The ability to perform this task endoscopically will vary with the skill and expertise of the surgeon. If the practitioner believes that the extent of the disease is too great, or if the likelihood of complications may increase due to performance of the procedure endoscopically, then it is appropriate to convert the procedure to laparotomy. This same form of decision-making process must be undertaken for large ectopic pregnancies and when complications or difficulties arise intraoperatively. Following salpingectomy for an ectopic pregnancy, approximately 40% of couples who desire to conceive achieve their goal, with a recurrent ectopic rate of approximately 20% (2).

Regardless of the mode of entry into the abdomen, in a patient with a large hemoperitoneum, the first step is to evacuate blood and blood clots so as to identify the site of bleeding. One method to accomplish this goal involves the introduction of a large-bore suction catheter for clot evacuation. In addition to devices specifically manufactured for suctioning (some of which are too narrow for use laparoscopically), the physician can use suction catheter tubing from which an end has been excised. Such tubing can be used either at an open procedure or laparoscopically by passage through a 10-mm trocar port.

Three major indications exist for extirpative procedures as opposed to conservative techniques such as salpingostomy (Table 7.2). The first is uncontrolled hemorrhage in which hemostasis cannot be achieved using conservative techniques. The most common cause is a ruptured ectopic, although such hemorrhage can also occur in ectopic pregnancies that are bleeding from the fimbriated end of the tube. In the latter case it may prove difficult to identify the source of bleeding and control it without causing extensive damage to the mucosal surfaces of the fallopian tube. In achieving hemostasis from a bleeding ectopic, it is important — to the extent possible — to minimize damage to the ipsilateral ovarian vasculature and ureter. This problem rarely occurs, except with ectopics that extend deeply into the mesosalpinx.

Importantly, unless damage has occurred to the ovarian vasculature, ipsilateral oophorectomy is unnecessary during treatment of an ectopic pregnancy by salpingectomy. For a woman who desires fertility, an oocyte derived from one ovary can potentially be picked up by the contralateral tube, thereby resulting in a pregnancy. Furthermore, in vitro fertilization and embryo transfer in these individuals may be possible at a later time

---

TABLE 7.2

**Indications for Extirpative
Surgery for Ectopic Pregnancies**

1. Uncontrolled hemorrhage
2. Nonrepairable tubal damage/distortion
3. Lack of desire for future fertility

should damage occur to the contralateral tube; in these cases, it would be advantageous to have as much ovarian tissue as possible.

The second occasion for performing a salpingectomy for an ectopic pregnancy involves a tube that is thought to be so severely damaged or distorted as to be nonrepairable. Unfortunately, it is not possible to give a precise description of when these conditions are met. Relative factors to be considered include the size of the ectopic, its location within the fallopian tube, the status of the tube (ruptured versus nonruptured), and, if ruptured, the size of the rent. Additional considerations include the presence of adhesions to the tube, the relation of the tube to nearby organs, and the status of the contralateral tube. In patients who desire fertility in whom the contralateral tube has already been removed, greater effort might be made to preserve the remaining fallopian tube. It must be remembered, however, that in a patient with both tubes, repeat ectopic pregnancies are just as likely to occur in a contralateral tube as an ipsilateral tube; thus no evidence appears to suggest that removal of the fallopian tube will reduce the patient's likelihood of developing a repeat ectopic pregnancy (3). A correlation to this observation would be the idea that tubal damage leading to ectopic pregnancy might follow from a process that involves both fallopian tubes.

A third indication for extirpative surgery for ectopic pregnancies involves patients who are certain that they do not desire future fertility. In such patients, it seems reasonable to perform a salpingectomy so as to minimize the likelihood of developing a repeat ectopic pregnancy in that fallopian tube. It must be emphasized, however, that no guarantee regarding elimination of ectopic pregnancies exists, as the patient might later develop an ectopic pregnancy in the intramural segment of the fallopian tube (which is not removed).

An additional consideration when contemplating extirpative surgery for ectopic pregnancy includes the location of the ectopic (4). For ampullary ectopic pregnancies, there now exist fairly strong data indicating that linear salpingostomy offers a high rate of success and is likely to result in tubes that heal without fistula formation or obstruction. In contrast, small series show that performance of linear salpingostomy for isthmic ectopic pregnancies is frequently (approximately 50%) followed by either fistula formation and/or tubal obstruction. This difference in outcome may reflect the different locations of the ectopics within the fallopian tube. In the ampullary segment, part or all of the eccyesis may actually appear between the tubal musculature and the serosa of the tube. In contrast, isthmic ectopic pregnancies are thought to be within the lumen of the tube themselves, in most cases.

Noting this divergence in histology, some surgeons have advocated segmental resection of isthmic ectopic pregnancies as a primary approach rather than salpingostomy. A qualified microsurgeon may be able to reanastomose the tube at that time, assuming that he or she can obtain the necessary instruments for microsurgical anastomosis. Because these tubes are often edematous and bleed relatively extensively, unlike in the performance of anastomosis on a nonpregnant patient, some would advocate delaying anastomosis to a later time. Although this decision seems reasonable, it necessitates that the patient undergo a subsequent operative procedure or, otherwise, leaves her with a fallopian tube segment that ends in a blind pouch. If the contralateral tube is patent, sperm could potentially enter the abdominal cavity from the contralateral side and be picked up along with an oocyte by this blind ending tube (5). This would set up a repeat ectopic pregnancy. Surprisingly, this type of event has been reported in the literature only a few times.

Taking into account these considerations, the author suggests attempting linear salpingostomy for isthmic ectopic pregnancies when possible, recognizing that there is an increased chance of obstruction or fistula development compared with an ampullary ectopic. If neither of these complications occurs, the patient will require no further surgical therapy. Alternatively, if a fistula develops or an obstruction occurs, a repeat surgical procedure with resection of this part of the tube and reanastomosis can be performed under controlled circumstances.

One final relative indication for performing an extirpative surgical procedure involves development of an ectopic in the cornual region of the tube. Such ectopics will frequently present at a later gestational age than ectopics in other locations throughout the fallopian tube. Consequently, they have often grown larger and may be embedded within the wall of the uterus. It is usually more difficult to obtain hemostasis in such cases, and treatment often relies on excision of a portion of the uterine tissue. Although conservative treatment of such ectopic pregnancies may, in some circumstances, be possible when the patient does not desire future fertility, the procedure will often cause extensive damage to the intramural portion of the fallopian tube. Consequently, it is rare for tubal patency to persist after these procedures on that side. If this treatment option would result in a blind ending tube, and if the patient planned to try to conceive using the contralateral tube, consideration should be given to removing the distal segment of the tube, thereby eliminating the possibility of developing an ectopic in this blind ending segment.

Once a salpingectomy has been selected as the surgical option, the surgeon must decide which modality to use. If undertaken at laparotomy, the first step in the most commonly performed procedure involves cross clamping the tube proximal to the site of the ectopic pregnancy and cross clamping the mesosalpinx so as to avoid the ovarian vasculature and the ureter. Avoidance of these other structures is usually easy, unless the patient has marked tissue distortion. This goal is best accomplished by placing clamps as close as possible to the tube itself. Depending on the size of the tube segment to be excised, the surgeon can address a varying number of pedicles. In each case, tissue is clamped, cut, and then tied using either free ties or stitch ligatures. Following excision of the tube, the surgeon should inspect the site for hemostasis. To the extent possible, blood clots in the abdominal cavity should be evacuated. The surgeon may choose to place an antiadhesion adjuvant in an attempt to minimize postoperative adhesion development. The author is unaware of any studies that have examined the efficacy of adjuvants in preventing adhesions to these sutured sites following salpingectomy.

Most surgeons tend not to perform extensive common surgical procedures at this time, because of the increased vascularity of the tissue and the lack of informed patient consent. Nonetheless, it is very much appropriate to explore the remainder of the pelvis, characterizing the extent of the disease to aid in future counseling of the patient.

Similar approaches are followed in ectopic pregnancies treated by salpingectomy at the time of laparoscopy, although the techniques should be modified based on the methods employed to achieve control of vascular pedicles (Table 7.3). The endoscopic procedures commonly involve two or three punctures. One puncture permits placement of the laparoscope at the umbilicus. Lower secondary trocar sites are placed either in the

TABLE 7.3

**Methods for Achieving Control of Pedicles
During Laparoscopic Salpingectomy**

Unipolar electrosurgery

Bipolar electrosurgery

Surgical clips

Linear cutters

Pretied suture loops

Laparoscopic suturing

Free sutures with intracorporeal or extracorporeal knotting

midline or to the sides. The location of these trocars will depend on surgeon preference. Some surgeons place two lower trocars, one on each side, so as to increase their separation and minimize their interference with one another. Another approach is to place one trocar in the midline, away from the epigastric vessels, so as to carry out diagnostic evaluation of the pelvis prior to determining the procedure that will be undertaken and the mode of access to be utilized. If the surgeon then decides to perform laparoscopic treatment, a third trocar can be placed ipsilateral to the tube with the ectopic pregnancy.

The author frequently elects to place a self-retaining grasping instrument through the port ipsilateral to the ectopic pregnancy. The tube is then grasped distal to the site of the ectopic pregnancy to allow manipulation. While the surgeon views the area through the laparoscope, an instrument can be placed through the remaining trocar sleeve to perform the procedure. In the case of extirpative surgery, the tube can be grasped approximately at the site of the ectopic. The tube and the underlying vascular arcade can then be coagulated.

Surgeons should be aware that the extent of electrosurgical damage will extend farther beyond the grasping instrument with unipolar electrosurgery than occurs with bipolar electrosurgery. These different tissue effects reflect the way in which these modalities work. With unipolar electrosurgery, the energy goes from the instrument through tissues, throughout the body, and back to the grounding plate. Thus divergence of energy occurs from the site where the energy source touches the tissue. In contrast, with bipolar electrosurgery, energy goes from one paddle of the instrument to the other, with most of the tissue damage confined to the area between these paddles. If bipolar instruments are used for longer periods of time, energy then does begin to diverge from the area of the paddles. Once the tissue has been adequately coagulated, the surgeon can excise it. He or she can use the electrosurgical instrument to grab along the mesosalpinx, performing a sequence of coagulation and cuttings so as to totally excise the eccyesis.

Many surgeons practice alternatives to electrosurgery, such as use of surgical clips, linear cutters, pretied surgical loops, and sutures as either free ties or stitch ligatures. Currently, no evidence indicates that any one of these modalities is preferable to the others. Instead, the choice will depend on the surgeon's preference and availability. Regardless of the method chosen, the physician should be appropriately trained and experienced in the use of that modality.

After excision of the tissue, a decision must then be made regarding how to remove it from the abdominal cavity. In most cases, this removal takes place through one of the trocar ports, as ectopic pregnancies are usually pliable. Care should be taken to minimize extrusion of the products of conception from the tissue being excised. If this extrusion does occur, the surgeon should grasp and remove the tissue. Although uncommon, implantation of such tissue following extrusion has occurred following laparoscopic salpingectomy. Consequently, it has been recommended that patients undergoing laparoscopic salpingectomies have repeat beta-hCG titers to rule out the presence of a persistent ectopic pregnancy, as is done for patients who undergo salpingectomy. These titers should be followed until they fall below the level of negativity for the assay.

In summary, extirpative surgical procedures for treatment of ectopic pregnancy are less frequently utilized than in the past, yet remain a reasonable option under many circumstances. Choice of the mode of entry into the abdominal cavity for salpingectomy, as for salpingostomy, will vary with a variety of factors — particularly, the experience of the surgeon and operating room personnel. The key consideration in making the surgical decision is the goal of providing the patient with the best possible care with the least risks of complications under the particular circumstances in which that patient presents.

REFERENCES

1. Doyle MB, DeCherney AH, Diamond MP. Epidemiology and etiology of ectopic pregnancy. In: Diamond MP, DeCherney AH, eds. Ectopic pregnancy: obstetrics and gynecology clinics of North America. Vol. 18. Philadelphia: WB Saunders, 1991:1–18.
2. Thornton KL, Diamond MP, DeCherney AH. Linear salpingostomy for ectopic pregnancy. In: Diamond MP, DeCherney AH, eds. Ectopic pregnancy: obstetrics and gynecology clinics of North America. Vol. 18. Philadelphia: WB Saunders, 1991:95–110.
3. DeCherney AH, Diamond MP. Laparoscopic salpingostomy for ectopic pregnancy. Obstet Gynecol 1987;70:948–950.
4. Diamond MP. Surgical aspects of infertility. In: Sciarra JJ, ed. Gynecology and obstetrics. Vol. 5. Philadelphia: Harper and Row, 1995:1–21.
5. Diamond MP, DeCherney AH. Distal segment tubal ectopic pregnancy after segmental resection for an isthmic ectopic. J Reprod Med 1988;33:236–237.

Reproductive Outcome After Treatment of Ectopic Pregnancy

Steven J. Ory

It has long been recognized that ectopic pregnancy may be a complication of infertility. Conversely, infertility often represents a sequela of ectopic pregnancy, even when the patient does not have preexisting infertility. A history of tubal damage — in particular, previous pelvic inflammatory disease — confers the highest relative risk for subsequent development of ectopic pregnancy; this history may also play a prominent role in infertility. Nevertheless, other factors unrelated to tubal disease — such as unexplained infertility, use of ovulation induction drugs, and assisted reproductive technologies — have also been noted to contribute independently to increased risk of ectopic pregnancy.

Reproductive performance following ectopic pregnancy is often the patient's primary concern. Although data describing pregnancy rates following treatment for tubal pregnancy go as far back as 50 years, they are limited and incomplete. In general, significant improvements in fertility outcome have been described over the past decades, but whether this trend reflects improved and earlier diagnosis, improved surgical technique, differences in populations studied, improved follow-up, or other unspecified causes remains unclear. All of these factors may play some role in confounding analysis of reproductive potential following ectopic pregnancy.

REPORTS PRIOR TO 1975

In 1955, Lund reported an extraordinary series of patients who were treated between 1930 and 1946 (1). Patients from three departments in a Copenhagen hospital were placed in two groups, with each group including more than 150 patients. All patients with the presumptive diagnosis of ectopic pregnancy (established via a positive Ascheim-Zondek or Friedman pregnancy test) were admitted for observation. The first group of patients — women with frank evidence of intra-abdominal hemorrhage and hypovolemia — were admitted to one of the three departments and underwent laparotomy and salpingectomy. The second group of patients were admitted to the other two departments and an attempt was made to manage them with bedrest alone; 57% were successfully managed without surgical intervention. In the entire series, only one fatality was reported, involving a postoperative bowel obstruction in one of the subjects managed surgically. The subsequent intrauterine pregnancy rate was 44% for the surgically treated patients and 46% for the nonsurgically treated subjects. The repeat ectopic pregnancy rate was 15% in both groups.

In 1962, Grant reviewed the experience of 353 women following salpingectomy for ectopic pregnancy (2). Only 22% of these patients subsequently delivered a live infant. Schenker et al evaluated 277 women treated for tubal pregnancy between 1955 and 1966 in six hospitals in Israel (3). Although 41% conceived after receiving treatment for an ectopic pregnancy, only 22% gave birth to one or more infants, and only 14% had recurrent ectopic pregnancies.

Jarvinen described one of the first experiences with conservative surgery, reviewing the experience of 30 patients treated conservatively between 1942 and 1952 at Helsinki University (4). In this series, 20 patients had the distal ampullary portion of their fallopian tubes removed (resection tubae); no successful pregnancies, one miscarriage, and one tubal pregnancy were experienced in these patients following this therapy. Seven patients had a linear salpingostomy (sectio tubae). Two women delivered successfully, one had a subsequent tubal pregnancy, and one experienced both a successful delivery and a spontaneous abortion. Three patients were treated with tubal expression of the embryo from the distal end of the tube (expressio ovi), and one of these patients had a successful pregnancy and spontaneous abortion. Several case reports of successful conservative surgery preceded Jarvinen's series.

Ploman and Wicksell reviewed the experience of 194 patients who underwent surgery for tubal pregnancy between 1944 and 1955 in Sweden (5). Of the 31 patients who had conservative surgery, 16 (52%) subsequently delivered a living child, 1 (3%) had a spontaneous abortion, and 5 (16%) had a subsequent tubal pregnancy. Of the 92 patients treated with extirpative surgery, 29 (32%) had a living child, 1 (1%) had a subsequent spontaneous abortion, and 6 (7%) had a subsequent tubal pregnancy.

Timonen and Niminen described a 10-year experience in Finland between 1954 and 1965, evaluating the fertility experience of 558 patients treated radically (with salpingectomy or salpingo-oophorectomy) and 185 patients treated conservatively (with tubal expression, salpingostomy, resection of the distal affected tube, or tubo-uterian implantation following resection) (6). Essentially no difference in the fertility rates was reported, with 29% of patients achieving term pregnancy after radical surgery and 27% experiencing term pregnancy after conservative surgery. The group treated with salpingostomy fared the best, with 30 (36%) of 83 patients achieving a term pregnancy. Recurrent extrauterine pregnancy occurred in 12% of the radically treated patients and 16% of the conservatively treated patients. Overall, 50% of the patients became pregnant after any type of surgery. The authors compared this experience with that of a series of patients treated earlier (between 1945 and 1951) at the same hospital, in which 39% of patients conceived.

REPORTED EXPERIENCE AFTER 1975

Reported pregnancy rates following surgical treatment of ectopic pregnancy improved significantly in the mid-1970s. The advent of microsurgical techniques developed in the late 1960s and their application in conservative procedures on the fallopian tube a few years later were cited as the likely causes for this trend. A number of other factors during the same period may have influenced fertility rates as well, however. For example, the increased prevalence of pelvic infections in the 1960s, the heightened awareness of their existence, and the broader availability of effective antibiotics for them permitted earlier intervention and may have served to minimize tubal damage.

In 1970, the Centers for Disease Control classified ectopic pregnancy as a reportable disease. Over the ensuing 20 years, the agency documented an exorbitant increase in the total number and incidence of ectopic pregnancy. Paradoxically, the mortality rate from ectopic pregnancy declined more than 90% during this same interval of time, suggesting that earlier diagnosis and intervention were occurring more often. The availability of very sensitive radioimmunoassays for human chorionic gonadotropin (hCG) capable of diagnosing more than 99% of pregnancies, the broad application of sonograms to exclude intrauterine pregnancies, and the more aggressive use of laparoscopy in the diagnosis and later treatment of ectopic pregnancy are the three technological advances usually credited with the earlier, more consistent, and ultimately more common diagnosis of ectopic pregnancy. Although conservative surgical procedures for ectopic pregnancy were widely embraced as contributing to improved fertility, appropriate studies comparing conservative to extirpative surgery were not conducted until later.

DeCherney reviewed a five-year experience with 98 patients treated between 1973 and 1977, in which 50 women underwent salpingectomy or salpingo-oophorectomy and 48 underwent salpingostomy (7). The viable pregnancy rate was 42% for the radically treated group and 40% for the conservatively treated group. The repeat ectopic rate was 10% for both groups. DeCherney concluded that no difference in outcomes was achieved with conservative versus radical surgery, but nevertheless recommended salpingostomy as the preferred treatment for unruptured ampullary ectopic pregnancy to preserve reproductive function.

Langer reported a series of 54 patients who underwent conservative surgical procedures in 1978 and 1979 (8). Following surgery, 80% of the patients developed an intrauterine pregnancy and 71% had a live birth. The recurrent tubal pregnancy rate was 12%. A group treated with radical surgery was not available for comparison.

In a more recent series (1972–1986), Langer reported the experience of 118 patients who underwent 149 conservative surgical procedures, including 116 cases of salpingostomy and 33 cases of tubal expression (9). The intrauterine pregnancy rate was 70% (83 of 118 patients) and the live birth rate was 64% (75 of 118 patients). Eleven percent experienced a recurrent tubal pregnancy, and none of the patients who underwent tubal expression had a recurrent ectopic pregnancy.

Hallatt reported the experience of 200 cases involving 1152 patients who underwent conservative surgery for ectopic pregnancy between 1953 and 1980 (10). Following surgery, 54% of the patients treated conservatively had an intrauterine pregnancy and 12% had a subsequent ectopic pregnancy. The repeat ectopic pregnancies were evenly distributed between the previously affected side and the contralateral side, leading the author to conclude that conservative surgery did not increase the subsequent risk of ectopic pregnancy. Fertility rates following salpingectomy from the same series were not described.

During approximately the same interval, Nagamani described 71 patients treated with salpingectomy or salpingo-oophorectomy in Texas (11). The conception rate with 3 to 13 years of follow-up was 62% and the recurrent ectopic rate was 13%. The study did not include patients who underwent conservative surgery.

Taken in the aggregate, these studies contributed to the notion that conservative surgery produced a superior fertility outcome. Nevertheless, few compared conservative to extirpative treatment in the same series, many reported total pregnancies rather than live-birth rates, and follow-up intervals were inconsistent.

MULTIFACTORIAL ANALYSES

More recent studies have analyzed multiple various risk factors for infertility following treatment of ectopic pregnancy and have provided some surprising results. Table 8.1 summarizes several studies describing fertility and repeat ectopic pregnancy rates after treatment for ectopic pregnancy, including analysis of risk factors. These data reveal a significant improvement in overall fertility as compared with earlier studies.

Surgical treatment does not appear to affect future fertility. For instance, a laparoscopic approach does not appear to influence subsequent

TABLE 8.1

Factors Affecting Fertility After Ectopic Pregnancy

Author, Year (Reference)	Age	Parity	Hx PID	Hx Infer-tility	Prior Ectopic	Type of Surgery	Adhesion/ Tubal Diseases	Number	Pregnancy (%)	Live Birth (%)	Ectopic (%)	Type of Surgery
Sherman, 1982 (12)	↓			↓		↑*	↓	47	83		6.4	Conservative
								104	72		5.8	Radical
Thorburn, 1988 (13)	↔		↔	↓	↓	↔						
Tuomivaara, 1988 (14)						↔		86	80		14	Conservative
								237	82		13	Radical
Mäkinen, 1989 (15)	↓	↔	↔			↔		42		69	29	Conservative
								68		63	15	Radical
Pouly, 1991 (16)	↔	↔	↓	↓	↓		↓					
Graft, 1994 (17)	↓				↓	↔	↓	44	52	27		Conservative
								71	52	32		Radical
Al-Nuaim, 1995 (18)	↓		↓	↓	↓							
Ory, 1993 (19)			↔	↓		↔		38	50		21	Conservative
								50	58		6	Radical

↑ = factor associated with improved fertility outcome; ↔ = no effect; ↓ = factor associated with worse fertility outcome; Hx = history of.
*Improved fertility associated with conservative surgery only for previously infertile patients.

reproductive outcome (23,24). Almost all of the studies conducted to date have compared fertility outcomes for patients treated with conservative procedures to those treated with extirpative procedures, finding no difference in subsequent fertility (12–15,17,19–22).

Clausen reviewed 40 studies published over a 40-year interval that evaluated the fertility prognosis after conservative and radical surgery for tubal pregnancy (21). This review included 7 studies describing conception rates after conservative surgery, 8 reporting conception rates after radical tubal surgery, 15 retrospective investigations comparing conservative to radical treatment, and 10 prospective selected treatment series. At the time of his review, no prospective, randomized investigations comparing radical to conservative surgery had been published. Clausen's review included a total of 4832 patients treated for ectopic pregnancy. Fourteen of the 15 retrospective studies comparing conservative and radical surgery found no difference in outcome. Likewise, Clausen concluded that a woman's risk of subsequent ectopic pregnancy did not increase after conservative surgery.

Perhaps the best measure of the efficacy of conservative surgery is fertility performance following conservative surgery for a single remaining fallopian tube. Oelsner et al reported the experience of 26 women who underwent conservative surgery on a single remaining fallopian tube (25). Forty-six percent subsequently had an intrauterine pregnancy, and 38.5% had a recurrent ectopic pregnancy. The number of successful pregnancies was not described, and the researchers did not note any difference between a macrosurgical or microsurgical technique. Valle and Lifchez reported on 13 patients over six years who received conservative surgery for a remaining tube. All 11 of the patients who subsequently attempted pregnancy achieved a successful vaginal delivery. Three experienced spontaneous abortions, and none had a subsequent ectopic pregnancy with 664 cumulative months of follow-up (26).

Infertility prior to treatment of ectopic pregnancy appears to be the strongest predictor of subsequent infertility (12,13,16,18–20). Studies in this area have cited significant differences in fertility prognosis between patients diagnosed with infertility prior to their ectopic pregnancy and those without such a diagnosis. This difference became even more obvious when patients were stratified for type of procedure (conservative versus radical) (19).

Increased age has generally been cited as a poor prognostic factor for future fertility (12,15,17,18), although not all studies have consistently identified such an association (13,16). The presence of pelvic adhesions and prior tubal disease has generally not signaled a poor prognosis (12,16,17). In addition, a prior history of pelvic inflammatory disease has not consistently been associated with poor fertility outcome, described as not influencing fertility potential by some authors (13,15,19) and decreasing fertility potential by others (16,18). Neither parity (15,16) nor the occurrence of postoperative complications (18) has been found to influence future fertility outcome. Although a single earlier report described reduced fertility potential following rupture of the affected tube (12), more recent studies have failed to observe an effect on subsequent fertility (13,16). Ectopic pregnancy occurring in conjunction with intrauterine device use was associated with a better fertility prognosis than failure to use such a device in three studies (13,27,28) but made no difference in a fourth study (15).

A prior ectopic pregnancy also consistently conveys a poor prognosis for successful intrauterine pregnancy; the prognosis becomes further compromised with each subsequent ectopic pregnancy (13,16–18,20). Glock et al reported the fertility experience of 37 patients who had at least two ectopic pregnancies between 1986 and 1989 (27). The intrauterine pregnancy rate among these women was 45%, but the live birth rate was only 27% and the recurrent ectopic pregnancy rate was 36%. Clausen reported an 11-year experience (from 1976 to 1987) of 50 women who desired pregnancy and were available for follow-up after surgical treatment of a second ectopic pregnancy with at least one remaining fallopian tube (28). Only 48% achieved any conception, 26% had at least one intrauterine pregnancy, and 32% experienced at least one additional ectopic pregnancy. Most other studies examining fertility after two ectopic pregnancies have noted a higher repeat ectopic pregnancy rate than intrauterine pregnancy rate and have described intrauterine pregnancy rates of less than 30% and lower successful pregnancy rates.

As noted previously, a woman's risk of incurring future ectopic pregnancy is increased after one ectopic pregnancy. In his extensive review of 40 studies, Clausen did not find any difference in subsequent risk between patients treated conservatively and radically (21). Although some authors have confirmed these findings (14,17), other studies have found a higher risk of ectopic pregnancy associated with conservative surgery (6,15,19).

CONCLUSIONS

Despite more than 50 years of reported experience, we still have an incomplete knowledge of fertility potential following ectopic pregnancy. It is clear that ectopic pregnancy has a significant effect on future fertility performance. This effect is particularly severe in patients who have had a prior diagnosis of infertility and who have experienced multiple ectopic pregnancies. These patients should be referred early for in vitro fertilization.

Although the current literature does not show any improvements in fertility outcomes for patients treated with conservative surgery rather than salpingectomy, the experience of utilizing conservative surgery for patients having a single remaining tube is encouraging and does support the notion that patients with conservatively treated fallopian tubes can subsequently conceive but may have a higher risk of future ectopic pregnancy. It is desirable to attempt to conserve a tube in patients desiring children when feasible, as radical surgery might be required in the future.

REFERENCES

1. Lund J. Early ectopic pregnancy: comments on conservative treatment. J Obstet Gynecol Br Emp 1955;62:70.
2. Grant A. The effect of ectopic pregnancy on fertility. Clin Obstet Gynecol 1962;5:861.
3. Schenker JG, Eyal F, Polishak WZ. Fertility after tubal pregnancy. Surg Gynecol Obstet 1972;135:74.
4. Jarvinen PA. Later fertility after conservative operation for tubal pregnancy. Ann Chir et Gyn Fenn 1954;43:185.
5. Ploman L, Wicksell F. Fertility after conservative surgery in tubal pregnancy. Acta Obstet Gynecol Scanda 1960;39:143.

6. Timonen S, Nieminen U. Tubal pregnancy: choice of operative method of treatment. Acta Obstet Gynecol Scand 1967;46:327.

7. DeCherney A, Kase N. The conservative surgical management of unruptured ectopic pregnancy. Obstet Gynecol 1979;54:451.

8. Langer R, Bukovsky I, Herman A, Sherman D, Sedovsky G, Caspi E. Conservative surgery for tubal pregnancy. Fertil Steril 1982;38:427.

9. Langer R, Raziel A, Ron-El R, Golan A, Bukovsky I, Caspi E. Reproductive outcome after conservative surgery for unruptured tubal pregnancy — a 15-year experience. Fertil Steril 1990;53:227.

10. Hallatt JG. Tubal conservation in ectopic pregnancy: a study of 200 cases. Am J Obstet Gynecol 1986;154:1216.

11. Nagamani M, London S, St. Amand P. Factors influencing fertility after ectopic pregnancy. Am J Obstet Gynecol 1984;149:533.

12. Sherman D, Langer R, Sadovsky G, Bukovsky I, Caspi E. Improved fertility following ectopic pregnancy. Fertil Steril 1982;37:497.

13. Thorburn J, Philipson M, Lindblom B. Fertility after ectopic pregnancy in relation to background factors and surgical treatment. Fertil Steril 1988;49:595.

14. Tuomivaara L, Kauppila A. Radical or conservative surgery for ectopic pregnancy? A follow-up study of fertility of 323 patients. Fertil Steril 1988;50:580.

15. Mäkinen JL, Salm TA, Nikkanen VPJ, Kaskinen EYJ. Encouraging rates of fertility after ectopic pregnancy. Int J Fertil 1989;34:46.

16. Pouly JL, Chapron C, Manhes H, Conis M, Wattiez A, Bruhat MA. Multifactorial analysis of fertility after conservative laparoscopic treatment of ectopic pregnancy in a series of 223 patients. Fertil Steril 1991;56:453.

17. Gruft L, Bertola E, Luchini L, Azzilonna C, Bigatti G, Parazzini F. Determinants of reproductive prognosis after ectopic pregnancy. Hum Reprod 1994;9:1333.

18. Al-Nuaim L, Bamgboye EA, Chowdbury N, Adelusi B. Reproductive potential after an ectopic pregnancy. Fertil Steril 1995;64:942.

19. Ory SJ, Nnadi E, Herrmann R, O'Brien PC, Melton LJ. Fertility following ectopic pregnancy. Fertil Steril 1993;60:231.

20. Querleu D, Boutteville C. Fertility after ectopic pregnancy. Fertil Steril 1989;51:1069.

21. Clausen I. Conservative versus radical surgery for tubal pregnancy. Acta Obstet Gynecol Scand 1996;75:8.

22. Menton M, Neeser E, Hirsch HA. Fertilität nach Tubargravidität: Vegleich von Tubenerhaltenden Operationen und Salpingektomien [Fertility after

tubal pregnancy: comparison of surgery preserving the fallopian tubes and salpingectomies] (in German with English abstract). Gebartsch Frauenheilk 1990;50:29.

23. Leindorff P, Thorburn J, Lindblom B. Fertility outcome after conservative surgical treatment of ectopic pregnancy evaluated in a randomized trial. Fertil Steril 1992;57:998.

24. Vermesh M, Presser SC. Reproductive outcome after linear salpingostomy for ectopic gestation: a prospective three-year follow-up. Fertil Steril 1992;57:682.

25. Oelsner G, Morad J, Carp H, Mashiach S, Serr DM. Reproductive performance following conservative microsurgical management of tubal pregnancy. Br J Obstet Gynecol 1982;94:1078.

26. Valle JA, Lifchez AS. Reproductive outcome following conservative surgery for tubal pregnancy in women with a single fallopian tube. Fertil Steril 1983;39:316.

27. Glock JL, Loy RA, Bramsted JR. Reproductive performance following a second ectopic gestation. Int J Gynecol Obstet 1993;43:191.

28. Clausen I Frost L, Børlum KG. Reproductive outcome following two ectopic gestatins: results after conservative surgery. Int J Fertil 1992;37:204.

29. Pouly JL, Chapron C, Conis M, Mage G, Wattiez A, Manhes H, Bruhat MA. Subsequent fertility for patients presenting with an ectopic pregnancy and having an intrauterine device in situ. Hum Reprod 1991;6:999.

30. Sandrei R, Ulstein M, Wollen A-L. Fertility following ectopic pregnancy with special reference to previous use of an intrauterine contraceptive device (IUCD). Acta Obstet Gynecol Scand 1987;66:131.

The Economic Impact of Ectopic Pregnancies

Scott Slayden
Ricardo Azziz

The use of cost analysis in the assessment of medical therapeutics has become integral to the goal of providing efficient and cost-effective medical services. In turn, the treatment of ectopic pregnancy (EP) and its sequelae represents a major burden to the health care system. For example, Washington and Katz estimated that the cost of treating EP in the United States amounted to $1.1 billion in 1990, with more than 88,000 women being affected (1). This figure probably underestimates the true cost, as these investigators considered only inpatient data. This chapter reviews the various diagnostic and therapeutic alternatives for the management of EP, emphasizing their cost-effectiveness.

COST ANALYSIS OF EP

Several resources are available to assist in the evaluation of the cost of any given disease process, including EP. Initially, a determination of the disease prevalence (or incidence) needs to be made. For EP, the U.S. Centers for Disease Control and Prevention (CDC) publishes relevant statistics (2). Information regarding hospitalized cases of EP can be derived from the CDC's National Hospital Discharge Survey (NHDS), and data regarding nonhospitalized cases of EP can be derived from the CDC's National

Hospital Ambulatory Care Survey (NHAMCS). Using these figures, the CDC estimated that EPs totaled 108,800 in 1992. Unfortunately, NHAMCS data can prove misleading, because several EP-related visits made by a single patient could be recorded inaccurately as several visits made by multiple patients. In addition, the NHAMCS database does not include patients examined and treated in physicians' offices with no direct hospital affiliation. These shortcomings, combined with the possibility of insufficient reporting of actual outpatient visits and geographical variations in EP prevalence, represent important areas of bias inherent in the NHAMCS database.

EP-related costs may be categorized into four general areas: 1) cost of diagnosis; 2) cost of treatment; 3) cost of treatment failure; and 4) indirect costs such as death, recurrent EP, lost wages, and future infertility. These costs are derived by analyzing several factors (Table 9.1). In this analysis, it is important to draw a distinction between hospital charges, provider reimbursement, and medical costs. Hospital charges may — but often do not — reflect the actual cost of providing a specific service. They typically are inflated 30% to 50% because of the frequent need for cost shifting among patients. In contrast, reimbursement varies widely and frequently amounts to 50% of the hospital charge. Under this scenario, the true cost of a given medical service would be difficult to calculate because charges and reimbursements represent the synthesis of diverse market pressures. Recognizing the difficulties in calculating true medical costs, the majority of studies have adopted hospital charges as a reflection of the cost of treatment.

COSTS OF DIAGNOSIS

Clearly, differences in the costs of diagnosing an EP depend on variances in the initial patient presentation, the diagnostic setting (for example, emergency room versus outpatient clinic), and the type, number, and accuracy of tests required to arrive at the diagnosis. When variations in the preceding factors are taken into consideration, it becomes clear that no single cost-effective diagnostic strategy is suitable for every case of suspected EP. Fortunately, enough similarities in initial patient presentation

TABLE 9.1

Potential Areas of Cost Incurred by the Surgical and Nonsurgical Treatment of Ectopic Pregnancy

Immediate Direct Medical Costs

Hospital Charges
- Daily accommodation fee × length of stay
- Operating room (utilization fee × operative time)
- Surgical equipment
- Anesthesia
- Laboratory
- Radiology
- Pharmacy
- Pathology
- Supplies

Professional Fees
- Nonsurgical (daily inpatient visits)
- Surgical

Outpatient Treatment and Followup
- Physician fees
- Laboratory fees
- Radiology (ultrasound fees)
- Pharmacy
- Supplies

Delayed Direct Medical Costs

Short-Term Sequelae
- Persistent ectopic pregnancy
- Complication rate (anemia, infection, ileus, and so on)

Future Sequelae
- Recurrent ectopic pregnancy
- Infertility evaluation and treatment
- Adhesive disease and chronic pelvic pain

Indirect Medical Costs

Physician training
Nursing training and utilization
Equipment purchase and depreciation

Indirect Nonmedical Costs

Lost wages
Lost productivity in the workplace
Sick leave benefits
Child care

exist to permit the development of generalized cost-effective diagnostic schemes. The following sections will focus on the costs associated with the diagnosis of EPs and comment on the more cost-effective strategies.

Initial Patient Presentation

In one study involving 161 women with an EP presenting to an emergency room (ER), only 2.5% patients required emergency surgery because of severe symptoms (3). These relatively rare patients with severe symptoms (such as hemodynamic instability) require a relatively inexpensive diagnostic evaluation, generally consisting of the initial ER visit and, at a minimum, a serum β-human chorionic gonadotropin (β-hCG) and a complete blood count (CBC). In some cases, however, their treatment is relatively expensive, taking the form of a laparotomy (discussed later in this chapter). Thus a low percentage of patients with EP undergo a very costly diagnostic procedure consisting of a laparotomy. When costs associated with a prolonged hospital stay, blood transfusions, hospital supplies and medications, lost wages, and prolonged recovery time are taken into consideration, the cost of treating patients who initially present with vascular instability becomes quite high. For example, at the authors' institution, representative charges and reimbursement (Blue Cross/Blue Shield rates for 1997) are $9500 and $6750, respectively.

In contrast to those patients presenting acutely, some 60% of patients visiting an ER for EP are "unruptured" and demonstrate minimal symptoms; another 38% are stable but considered to be ruptured with clinical evidence of intra-abdominal bleeding (3). Finally, many patients are not seen initially in the ER but rather diagnosed before the onset of significant symptoms. In these less acute cases, the goal of the diagnostic evaluation is to avoid costly surgical intervention and hospitalization, while maximizing diagnostic accuracy, preventing EP rupture, and avoiding hemodynamic collapse, as discussed below.

Setting

It is generally assumed that a visit to the ER costs more than a typical outpatient visit. For example, 1996 charges at the authors' institution for a theoretical four-hour patient visit to the ER to evaluate for EP totaled $622. This charge includes a triage fee ($75), observation fee

($50/hour), transvaginal ultrasound ($231), CBC ($28), and urinary ($37) and quantitative serum β-hCG ($50) determinations. These charges may be compared with the costs for a similar encounter in an outpatient clinic setting, which totals $503: new-patient extended evaluation ($200), ultrasound ($200), CBC ($28), and urinary ($25) and serum quantitative β-hCG ($50) determinations. In this setting, a savings of 18% ($118) was realized by evaluating a stable patient with a suspected EP in an outpatient clinic setting. Alternatively, if the ER visit required only two hours' time, the cost difference would be only $18.

Nonetheless, many patients seen in an outpatient clinic do not represent a new-patient visit and would be charged only for an extended return visit ($90 charge). Stovall et al noted that 45% of women with an EP initially evaluated in an ER had a benign clinical presentation and could have been evaluated in an outpatient clinic (3).

Tests

The cost and complexity of tests used to assist in the diagnosis of EP range from the simple and inexpensive urinary hCG determination to the relatively costly laparoscopy. The decision to employ any or all of the available diagnostic tests is influenced significantly by the patient's clinical presentation. Consequently, several generalized diagnostic schemes may be developed for similar groups of patients. For example, different diagnostic schemes may take into account the patient's desire to maintain her current pregnancy and future fertility, her initial hemodynamic stability, or previous medical history. The remainder of this section will review the cost-effectiveness of several commonly used basic (that is, urinary and serum β-hCG, serum progesterone [P4] levels, and ultrasonography) and advanced diagnostic tests (that is, laparoscopy, uterine dilatation and curettage [D&C], and culdocentesis).

Basic Diagnostic Tests: The minimal initial laboratory evaluation of a woman complaining of amenorrhea, abnormal vaginal bleeding, and/or pelvic pain should include a qualitative *urinary hCG test*. Current qualitative hCG immunoassays have more than adequate sensitivity (25 to 50 mIU/mL, first international reference preparation [IRP]) and rapidity (2 to 5 minutes), yet cost less than serum β-hCG measurement (for example, \$37 versus \$50 at our institution, respectively). Thus the urinary hCG test may serve as the front-line screen in patients with a suspected EP.

If the qualitative pregnancy test is positive, a *transvaginal ultrasound (TVUS)* should be obtained in symptomatic patients and patients with EP risk factors. Transvaginal ultrasonography has supplanted transabdominal sonography and is frequently used in the initial evaluation of patients with a suspected EP. Demonstration of a normal intrauterine pregnancy (IUP) generally is associated with the absence of an EP, except in the rare case of heterotopic pregnancies. Alternatively, visualization of fetal cardiac activity in the adnexa, which occurs in approximately 9% of all EPs, confirms the diagnosis of EP and mandates immediate therapy (4).

In some cases, serial sonography may prove helpful in establishing the diagnosis of an EP. Cacciatore et al used serial weekly TVUS in 225 asymptomatic patients at high risk for this disorder, of which 55 (24.4%) actually had an EP (5). Of the remaining patients, 30 (13.3%) had miscarriages and 140 (62.2%) had a continuing IUP. Eighty-four percent of EPs were diagnosed at the initial sonogram, at a median gestational age of 37 days. All remaining patients with an EP were diagnosed within the next seven days at repeat sonography, with 4 of 9 developing mild symptoms during this time. Thus early use of TVUS may enable identification of an EP prior to the development of symptoms, allowing for early and less costly intervention.

More recently, the addition of color Doppler flow analysis at TVUS has been shown to improve the diagnostic sensitivity of this imaging modality in some patients, although its cost-effectiveness (and accuracy) remain to be determined (6).

If the initial sonography fails to detect an IUP or EP, a *single serum quantitative β-hCG* should be obtained. Recommendations for therapy or follow-up may be based on the results of this single test, considering the findings at the initial sonography and the patient's presenting symptoms. For example, if the β-hCG level exceeds 1500 mIU/mL (first IRP), TVUS fails to detect an IUP US, and the patient has minimal symptoms, consideration should be given to proceeding directly to therapy, particularly in patients not wishing to preserve the pregnancy (7). Nonetheless, most physicians are reluctant to base their therapy or diagnosis on a single laboratory method, which may be subject to a significant risk for human and/or technical error. Furthermore, the majority of patients with an EP (58% to 91%) demonstrate an initial β-hCG level of less than 1000 mIU/mL during their initial evaluation, at which point TVUS would not be expected to visualize an IUP (8).

The use of *serial serum β-hCG determinations* (once every 48 hours) is a well-established method for determining the viability of a pregnancy, although the cost-effectiveness of this scheme remains unclear. In fact, Shepherd et al have demonstrated that this method of follow-up is less useful (and probably not cost-effective) when screening asymptomatic patients at risk for having an EP (9).

In addition to hCG determinations and ultrasonography, measurement of *a single serum P4 level* has been employed as an initial laboratory test to determine the viability of an early pregnancy. Despite the fact that a significant number of studies have examined the use of P4 measures in the evaluation of abnormal early gestation, only a small number of physicians appear to use this test.

Stovall has suggested using the serum P4 assay in the initial phases of an algorithm for the diagnosis and treatment of EP (10). In his study, 97% of patients with a completed abortion and 56% of patients with an EP had a P4 of less than 5.0 ng/mL at the time of diagnosis. In fact, a P4 of less than 5.0 ng/mL was generally associated with the absence of a normal gestation of any type, allowing for immediate, more cost-effective therapy to be provided. In contrast, a P4 value exceeding 25 ng/mL was strongly suggestive of a normal pregnancy and could be used to prevent costly intervention, with only 1.6% of patients with an EP and 4.2% with a failing IUP having a P4 level higher than this value. Unfortunately, 44% of EP patients had a P4 level between 5.0 ng/mL and 25 ng/mL at their initial presentation, severely limiting the usefulness of this assay.

The use of a P4 measurement in the more than 60% of all U.S. patients with an EP who demonstrate minimal symptoms at their initial presentation would result in an additional national annual expenditure of $2.6 million (calculated at an institutional charge of $40 per assay). Nonetheless, the proposed advantages of a more rapid diagnosis (by approximately 24 hours) and a lower risk of rupture remain to be confirmed.

Advanced Diagnostic Tests: As noted earlier, in many patients who are at risk for an EP the diagnosis is not established with reasonable certainty at the initial evaluation. Nonetheless, if the patient does not wish to maintain the pregnancy, an *immediate D&C* may be performed. Demonstration of chorionic villi in the curettage specimen effectively excludes an EP in the majority of cases and may reduce the need for costly follow-up visits. Alternatively, if villi are not identified, immediate medical therapy for an EP (discussed later in this chapter) may be instituted to avoid the higher costs and morbidity associated with intra-abdominal hemorrhage.

Despite these theoretical benefits, the utilization of a diagnostic/therapeutic D&C in the evaluation of EP has not been assessed from a cost-analysis perspective. The costs of such a procedure will vary widely, depending on the operative setting, type of anesthesia used, and pathologic services requested. For example, the charges for a D&C performed in a hospital operating room (OR) at the authors' institution amount to approximately $5081 (physician's fee, $650; OR, $2777; anesthesia, $763; pharmacy, $327; recovery room, $126; postoperative respiratory care, $108; and pathology, $330). In contrast, charges for a D&C performed in our outpatient surgical center are $2156, or $2925 less than the cost of the same procedure performed in the hospital OR.

The gestational age at initial presentation for most patients with an EP is less than seven menstrual weeks. If this early gestational age is taken into consideration, many patients with a suspected EP may qualify for an office suction curettage (for example, menstrual extraction) with minimum cervical dilatation. The technique of "menstrual extraction" performed before seven weeks' gestation, pioneered in the early 1970s, has a 95% to 97% rate of successful IUP evacuation (11,12). This technique may prove to be a much more cost-effective method of uterine evacuation and diagnosis in many patients with a suspected EP. The charges at our institution approximate $577, which is $2348 and $4500 less than the comparable outpatient surgical center and hospital OR charges, respectively.

A final point to be considered when performing a diagnostic D&C is the use of frozen section specimen analysis, as this test doubles the total pathology fee (to more than $600 at our institution). Frozen sections should be used sparingly.

In 40% of patients with an EP, a *laparoscopy* may potentially serve as the ultimate diagnostic tool. This method of diagnosis offers the advantage of allowing simultaneous therapy to be performed. It has the disadvantage of high cost, ranging from $5000 to $7000. Nonetheless, diagnostic/operative laparoscopy may ultimately prove to be cost-effective in some cardiovascularly stable patients, as indicated later in this chapter.

Finally, *culdocentesis* has lost favor as a diagnostic modality for EP. Indeed, the utility of this method has diminished as the ability of ultrasound to detect small amounts of cul-de-sac fluid has improved. A positive culdocentesis merely confirms the presence of a hemoperitoneum without establishing the source (13,14). Thus, in most patients, culdocentesis appears to add unnecessary costs and morbidity to the diagnosis of EP.

COSTS OF TREATMENT

The three general treatment regimens for EP involve surgery, medical therapy, and expectant management. The clinical situation and care provider experience generally will dictate the selection of a treatment modality. An improvement in early diagnosis, as well as physician awareness of risk predictors and therapeutic options, will serve to lower the cost of EP treatment.

Surgical Costs

Traditionally, EP has been a surgically treated disease. A significant number of studies have evaluated the cost-effectiveness of various surgical modalities — principally, operative laparoscopy versus laparotomy. Despite the fact that few of these reports have determined the actual cost-effectiveness of the treatment protocol undergoing evaluation, a certain degree of savings may be inferred from their results. Using 1987 CDC estimates of EP incidence, Azziz and Maruri calculated an overall national savings of $138 million per year (in 1982 dollars), if 80% of EPs were treated with operative laparoscopy as opposed to laparotomy (15). Other studies (Table 9.2) indicate that operative laparoscopy saves an average of $1350 per case when compared to laparotomy, with laparoscopy patients returning to work on average 2.9 weeks faster than laparotomy patients

TABLE 9.2

Economic Advantages of Laparoscopy (LSC) Versus Laparotomy (LAP)

Study	Year	Number of Patients	Outcome	Overall Savings of LSC
Gray et al (16)	1995	109	LSC: 16-minute reduction in operating time, 3-day reduction in hospital stay, 19% required medical/surgical intervention for persistent trophoblast. LAP: Similar recovery time to LSC. 5% required second medical or surgical intervention.	LSC: 40% less expensive than LAP.
Maruri, Azziz (15)	1993	Approximately 70,400	LSC: LSC applicable to approximately 80% of 88,000 ectopic pregnancies in 1987 (representing 77,400 cases). Hospital savings of $1500 per LSC case and return to work 17 days faster per LSC case.	LSC: Savings of $136 million per year in hospital charges, lost wages, and home care.
Murphy et al (17)	1992	62	LSC: Significant reduction in postoperative hospital stay and return to work; 11% required further surgery or MTX. LAP: Similar operative times.	LSC: $1200 in hospital charges saved per case.
Baumann et al (18)	1991	87	LSC: 3.5-day shorter hospital stay. 1.8-week faster return to domestic activities. 3.2-week faster return to work. LAP: Similar operating time as LSC.	LSC: 50% less expensive than LAP.
Vermesh et al (19)	1989	60	LSC: $1500 savings/case due to shortened hospital stay. LAP: Longer recovery time. Persistent trophoblast, tubal patency, and future IUP rates similar to LSC.	LSC: $1500 savings per case in hospital charges only.

TABLE 9.2

(*continued*)

Study	Year	Number of Patients	Outcome	Overall Savings of LSC
Erny, Campio-Budar (20)	1989	109	LSC: Reduced hospital stay by 4.2 days. Reduced work leave by 22 days.	LSC: Saved FF8954/case.
Levine (21)	1985	21	LSC: Mean postoperative hospital stay for any type of LSC surgery was 0.5 to 2.0 days. LAP: Mean postoperative stay for matched LAP procedures was 5.0 to 5.7 days.	LSC: Saved 49% per case in hospital costs.

(16–21). Although linear salpingostomy is a conservative procedure with a possible greater chance of persistent EP (22), there does not appear to be a significant difference in operative time, retained trophoblastic tissue, operative and postoperative complications, or subsequent fertility rates when laparotomy and laparoscopy are compared in a randomized prospective fashion (19).

Despite known savings in cost and convalescence time, evidence suggests that operative laparoscopy remains underutilized as a treatment for EP (23). The reasons for this finding probably are related to the fact that this surgical technique is a relatively recent development, with the first EP to be treated laparoscopically being reported in 1973 (24). Only in the mid-1980s did rapid development and teaching of advanced laparoscopic techniques occur. Thus a significant number of physicians who were trained prior to this time continue to perform laparotomies to treat EPs.

Although medical treatment may be more cost-effective than surgery in many patients with an EP (see below), operative laparoscopy remains most useful in cardiovascularly stable patients who meet one of the following criteria:

- They desire permanent sterilization.
- They develop an EP secondary to sterilization failure and require immediate treatment.
- They require immediate treatment, but not an emergency laparotomy.
- They have an unclear diagnosis.

Laparotomy should be reserved for the few patients (4%) who are vascularly unstable and require immediate treatment.

Mini-laparotomy

A potential alternative to laparoscopy is the treatment of EP via an outpatient mini-laparotomy. This surgical technique may be employed in areas underserved by skilled laparoscopists to produce significant savings in terms of reduced hospital costs without appreciably altering patient outcome or satisfaction. Alternatively, mini-laparotomy may be used in cases of EP that are unsuitable for laparoscopic treatment based on preoperative or intraoperative findings, but that do not require a laparotomy. Several studies have demonstrated that this strategy can significantly reduce hospital stays (generally less than 24 hours) and is safe, effective, and economical (Table 9.3).

Medical Therapy

The tradition of surgical therapy for EPs changed in 1982 with the report by Tanaka et al of the successful medical treatment of an unruptured cornual pregnancy with intramuscular (IM) methotrexate (MTX) injection (29). Since then, various groups have reported the medical management of EP, including the following regimens:

- The injection of MTX, hypertonic saline, hyperosmolar glucose, or prostaglandin directly into the EP
- Multiple-dose IM MTX with or without leucovorin rescue
- Single-dose IM MTX

Stovall et al have demonstrated that a single-dose IM MTX protocol is superior to other MTX delivery routes in terms of toxicity and offers similar success rates (30).

TABLE 9.3

Short-Stay Laparotomy and Mini-laparotomy

STUDY	YEAR	NUMBER OF PATIENTS	OUTCOME	OVERALL SAVINGS
Berger (25)	1994	373	373 patients underwent laparotomy for various gynecologic indications; 98% had no complications, and 99% required no hospitalization.	Not calculated
Fayez, Dempsey (26)	1993	484	484 patients underwent elective gynecologic surgery via laparotomy with hospital discharge after overnight stay. No immediate or late postoperative complications were noted, and no rehospitalizations occurred.	Not calculated
Silva et al (27)	1991	17	17 tubal reanastomosis cases performed with combined LSC/mini-laparotomy technique were compared with 5 cases performed with standard LAP technique. Of 17 study patients, 15 were managed as outpatients with no observed complications. Return to work was 17 days sooner in the mini-laparotomy group.	$2603 saved per mini-laparotomy case
Loffer (28)	1987	23	17 of 23 patients had a mini-laparotomy incision. Of these patients, 11 were managed as outpatients and the other 6 were discharged after an overnight hospital stay. No complications of outpatient management were noted.	Not calculated

The economic advantage of IM MTX injection compared with laparoscopy in selected cases is readily evident (Table 9.4). Alexander et al reviewed the literature and compared the reimbursement associated with the use of IM MTX, laparoscopy, and laparotomy in treating small unruptured EPs (31). In their example, the MTX treatment strategy would

TABLE 9.4

Economic Advantages of Methotrexate (MTX) Versus Surgery for Treatment of Ectopic Pregnancy

Study	Year	Number of Patients	Outcome	Overall Savings of MTX
Alexander et al (31)	1996	N/A	MTX: Reimbursement range = \$438–\$1390. Saving = \$1124–\$2536 over LSC. LSC: Reimbursement range = \$2506 – \$2904.	MTX used in 45% of 88,000 ectopics would save \$43–\$97 million/year.
Stovall et al (32)	1994	60	MTX: Mean cost of single-dose MTX was \$1563. No treatment failures or significant side effects were noted. LSC: Mean cost was \$6626 with a mean hospital stay of 2.5 days and no persistent trophoblast. One patient experienced a major postoperative complication. LAP: Mean charges were \$8001 with a mean length of stay of 5.2 days. All patients had one or more postoperative complications.	MTX saved \$5063 compared to LSC and \$6438 compared to LAP.

TABLE 9.4

(*continued*)

Study	Year	Number of Patients	Outcome	Overall Savings of MTX
Creinin et al (33)	1993	50	MTX: 50 consecutive cases of ectopic pregnancy were reviewed. 30% were eligible for MTX treatment, with an estimated cost savings of $160,000. The study did not evaluate outpatient cases.	$280 million would be saved annually in the United States if 30% of 88,400 cases were treated with MTX.

need to have a dismal 15% success rate before laparoscopy became more cost-effective than this regimen. In their estimation, even at the lowest reported success rate of 58%, MTX therapy would cost $1124 less than an ideal 100% successful laparoscopic salpingostomy (Table 9.5). These savings take into account the unusual patient who requires overnight hospital admission after MTX injection or repeat IM MTX injection for persistent EP.

In an effort to estimate the cost savings of MTX therapy, Stovall utilized institutional charge data for ER visits, office visits, laboratory, pharmacy, and ultrasound services to determine the average cost associated with the single-dose IM MTX protocol for treating EP in 21 patients (32). The average total charges for MTX therapy per EP patient amounted to $1563, representing an average savings of $5063 and $6438 over laparoscopy and laparotomy, respectively. Creinin et al estimated that approximately 30% to 45% of all EPs in the United States could qualify for this treatment. Based on these data, annual savings of $43 million to $280 million have been calculated (31,32).

TABLE 9.5

Cost for Treatment Components of Different Management Strategies for the Small Unruptured Ectopic Pregnancy

TREATMENT	INCLUDES	COST ($)
Methotrexate, one dose	Medication	5
	Laboratory	25
	Follow-up	409
	Total	**439**
Methotrexate, repeat dose	Medication	5
	Laboratory	40
	Follow-up	103
	Total	**148**
Laparoscopy	OR time	1250
	Surgeon fees	800
	Anesthesia	350
	Laboratory	15
	Pathology	27
	Follow-up	64
	Total	**2506**
23-hour observation	**Total**	**380**
Laparotomy	OR time	820
	Surgeon fees	800
	Anesthesia	350
	Laboratory	15
	Hospitalization	1080
	Follow-up (2 visits)	113
	Pathology	27
	Total	**3205**

SOURCE: Reprinted with permission of the American College of Obstetricians and Gynecologists. From: Treatment of the small unruptured ectopic pregnancy: a cost analysis of methotrexate versus laparoscopy. Obstet Gynecol 1996;88:123–127.

These data support the cost-efficacy of a single IM injection of MTX in treating EP and provide strong support for the recommendation of this technique as the primary treatment modality for many small, unruptured EPs.

Expectant Management

Another potential area of cost savings may lie in the expectant management of selected EPs (Table 9.6). The goal of this management strategy is to lower costs and morbidity by predicting which EPs will resolve spontaneously without requiring medical or surgical intervention.

In a prospective study, Trio et al evaluated 112 patients suspected to have an EP and selected 67 (60%) patients to be managed expectantly (34). Initial selection criteria for these patients were the absence of hemodynamic instability, lack of abdominal pain, ultrasound evidence of free peritoneal fluid of more than 100 mL, adnexal mass greater than 4 cm, or embryonic heartbeat. Forty-nine (73%) patients achieved a spontaneous resolution, and the remainder required therapy (three received medical treatment and the remaining underwent surgery). The researchers noted that an initial β-hCG titer of less than 1000 mIU/mL predicted resolution in 88% of patients. As determined by the β-hCG titer, the mean time to resolution in patients successfully managed expectantly was similar to that following treatment with IM MTX (31 $\pm$ 19 days versus 35.5 $\pm$ 11.8 days, respectively).

A study by Ylostalo et al produced similar results (8); spontaneous resolution was observed in 57 (69%) of 83 patients followed expectantly, and the remainder required laparoscopic surgery. Selection criteria for expectant management in this study included decreasing levels of serum β-hCG, EP diameter less than 4 cm on TVUS, and no clinical intra-abdominal signs. Among 318 patients evaluated, 83 (26%) met these criteria.

The major economic disadvantage associated with expectant management of asymptomatic EP is related to the relatively high failure rate (20% to 30%) and the cost associated with the follow-up visits, sonograms, and β-hCG determinations. Several reports, however, indicate that many patients undergoing surgery after failed expectant management may have qualified for MTX treatment as a means of resolving the EP at a reduced cost. Thus

TABLE 9.6

Expectant Management of Ectopic Pregnancy

Study	Year	Number of Patients	Outcome	Overall Savings
Trio et al (33)	1995	67	67 of 112 patients qualified for expectant management. Spontaneous resolution occurred in 73%, 22% required surgery, and 4% required medical therapy.	Not calculated
Ylostalo et al (10)	1992	318	83 of 318 patients qualified for expectant management. Spontaneous resolution occurred in 69%, and 31% required surgery.	Not calculated
Mayman et al (34)	1992	81	Meta-analysis from 8 studies. 76% resolved spontaneously, and 24% required surgery.	Not calculated
Kooi and Kock (35)	1992	74	Meta-analysis from 7 studies. 78% resolved spontaneously, and 12% required surgery.	Not calculated
Garcia et al (36)	1987	13	1 of 13 patients (8%) required surgery.	Not calculated

the low cost and minimal risk associated with primary MTX treatment require consideration in these early asymptomatic cases. A randomized prospective study is needed to compare the outcome and cost-effectiveness of expectant management with MTX in similar patients with an EP.

Treatment Failures

Treatment failure increases the overall cost associated with EP. Nevertheless, treatment failure is often unavoidable for two reasons: the patient usually prefers to undergo conservative therapy so as to preserve her future fertility, or use of the least invasive and costly method of therapy (for example, laparoscopic surgery or MTX therapy) may be mandated. The rate of treatment failure depends on the type of therapy rendered, the clinical presentation, and provider experience. The cost of treating these failures is influenced by the choice of laparoscopy, laparotomy, or MTX as the second therapy.

Fortunately, the overall rate of treatment failure is low. Indeed, it is virtually nil when the patient undergoes a salpingectomy, either laparoscopically or via laparotomy. When conservative therapeutic options are selected (laparoscopic salpingostomy and IM MTX injection), treatment failure may be a more common and variable event. The study by Alexander et al (31) considers the significant variability of treatment failure rates seen with laparoscopy (ranging from 0% to 17%) and MTX therapy (6% to 28%) in comparing the cost-effectiveness of these treatment modalities. Including the cost of treatment failures and combining the worst-case scenario for MTX therapy (that is, a failure rate of 28%) with the best outcome reported for laparoscopy (that is, a failure rate of 0%), the MTX treatment option remained $1124 less expensive than laparoscopy when repeat MTX was used to treat those failures.

Using these data and assuming that 45% of patients with an EP are eligible for either laparoscopy or MTX therapy, both of which have a hypothetical failure rate of 15%, $3.2 million per year would be spent treating EP failures in the United States if MTX were the sole treatment option (108,800 EP/year × 0.45 × 0.15 × $439 = $3,224,016) and $18.4 million per year would be spent treating failures if laparoscopy were the sole treatment option (108,800 EP/year × 0.45 × 0.15 × $2506/laparoscopy = $18,404,064).

INDIRECT COSTS OF EP

Lost Wages

In addition to those costs directly associated with medical care, indirect costs should be considered when assessing the economic impact of EP. For example, using 1989 data from the U.S. Bureau of Labor and CDC, Azziz and Maruri estimated the national annual value of lost wages associated with the laparoscopic treatment of hospitalized cases of EP to be $64,931,925 (15). Approximately 108,800 cases of EP occurred in 1992 (combining the NHCAMS and NHDS data). According to 1995 Bureau of Labor statistics, 71% of noninstitutionalized women (aged 16 to 44 years) are employed, at a median weekly salary of $450, or $90/workday (38). If we assume that 10% of patients are treated medically, 50% undergo laparoscopy, and the remainder receive a laparotomy, and that the mean convalescence is 3.0 days, 6.7 days, and 25 days with these therapies, respectively (39), then the annual cost of lost wages amounts to more than $96 million annually. Alternatively, treating 25% of patients medically, 60% laparoscopically, and the remainder via laparotomy would save more than $36 million annually in lost wages. Overall, these monies represent either lost earnings to the patient (if she does not receive sick pay) or lost income to her employer (if she does qualify for this benefit).

Child or Home Care Costs

It is difficult to calculate the monies expended in caring for the patient and/or her children during her postoperative recuperation time. As previously noted, patients undergoing laparotomy surgery for an EP require an average of 17 more days to "return to normal activity" than patients undergoing laparoscopic surgery (39). Because these patients are mostly of reproductive age, many probably have young children who require additional care while their mother is recuperating from surgery. Unfortunately, the exact extent of this problem cannot be quantified with present data.

Patient Deaths

The highest single cost associated with an EP relates to the death of a patient. Fortunately, death from EP is a rare event, with 3.8 deaths per

10,000 EP reported in 1988 (40). If this rate is extrapolated to the latest statistics of 108,800 EP per year, then 41 deaths will be predicted to occur.

In a theoretical example, if a 20-year-old woman working 44 weeks per year at the mean age-adjusted 1995 U.S. weekly salary of $406 died as a result of an EP, the estimated minimum lost future wages would be $625,000 if she had retired at the age of 55 and annual wage increases are not taken into account. In addition, her tax contributions over these years would be lost. Although these calculations cannot begin to estimate the emotional toll of a human death, they do serve to highlight yet another area of economic loss associated with EP.

Treatment of Associated Infertility

Another area of cost associated with EP is the diagnosis and treatment of related infertility. In the best-case scenario, approximately 20% of women diagnosed with an EP will experience subsequent infertility (41) secondary to tubal disease. Using 1992 CDC figures, we can estimate that 21,760 patients will experience such infertility, although only 43% (9357 patients) will likely seek care for their problem (42). Assuming that IVF is utilized in all patients seeking infertility care at an average 1992 cost of $8000 (43), a potential expenditure of more than $148 million would be required for the performance of two IVF treatment cycles in these individuals. Of course, many of these infertile patients will be unable to afford even one IVF treatment cycle, and many others will resort to costly tubal surgery.

Recurrent EP

After experiencing an EP, a patient's risk of developing a recurrent EP increases from approximately 1% to 2% before the event to 10% to 30% after the EP (44–47). Washington and Katz did not calculate the costs of treating recurrent EP. Nonetheless, the estimated average repeat EP rate of 10% would be associated with a very significant expenditure in health care dollars. From the estimated 108,800 yearly pool of EP patients in 1992, 10,880 (10%) women would experience a repeat EP. It is assumed the majority of these women would undergo surgical therapy, and reimbursement data from the study of Alexander et al may therefore be used to estimate these costs (31). If the least expensive surgical alternative of operative laparoscopy were employed in 80% of these EPs (that is, in 8704 cases) at a reimbursable cost of $2506 per case, a total additional expenditure of more than $21 million would result. Replacing laparoscopy with a single dose of MTX in only half of these cases would save nearly $9 million.

CONCLUSION

The cost-effective treatment of EP demands an early diagnosis before tubal rupture, knowledge of both medical and surgical therapeutic alternatives, patient compliance, and a desire to use MTX in appropriate clinical situations. The diagnosis of EP at an early stage may provide the greatest cost savings through prevention of morbid sequelae and avoidance of expensive surgical therapy.

Patients at high risk for developing EP should be screened with a urine hCG test and TVUS early during their fifth week of gestation. Each physician should have a clear idea of his or her own hCG discriminatory zone, above which a normal IUP is always seen with TVUS. In patients with a known menstrual history, the absence of a gestational sac — particularly by six weeks' gestation — should prompt serum quantitative hCG determinations. On the other hand, hCG and TVUS screening of asymptomatic low-risk individuals does not appear to be cost-effective.

In addition to possible savings associated with early diagnosis through screening of high-risk individuals, a great deal of money may be saved through the use of MTX therapy instead of surgery (that is, laparoscopy, laparotomy, and/or D&C). Furthermore, if surgery is considered, it should be carried out in a low-cost setting. Certainly, the cost-effectiveness and risks associated with MTX therapy versus those linked to expectant management of patients with suspected EP needs to be compared, although there currently is little enthusiasm for the latter form of therapy, given its greater associated patient anxiety, prolonged follow-up, and litigation risk.

To realize continued savings in both treatment costs and convalescence time, every effort must be made to focus on the prevention and early diagnosis of EP. Prevention should be effected by targeting young women with educational programs that highlight the negative impact of EP on future fertility and its associated morbidity. Most adolescent females seem to be unaware of this association, yet may be keenly aware of the importance of protecting their reproductive capabilities. In addition, a conscious effort must be made among women's health care providers to identify and educate their patients who are at risk of developing an EP.

Unfortunately, the group of patients identified as having the highest risk of EP are those who receive the most discontinuous health care. In these patients, prevention of a repeat EP may be a more attainable goal if time is taken to explain the importance of returning early upon suspicion of pregnancy and to stress that early diagnosis may avoid surgery. Equally important is the need for providers to become facile in methods of diagnosing EP during the interval most responsive to medical management and to obtain training in the appropriate use of MTX.

REFERENCES

1. Washington AE, Katz P. Ectopic pregnancy in the United States: economic consequences and payment source trends. Obstet Gynecol 1993;81:287–292.
2. Center for Disease Control. Ectopic pregnancy — United States, 1990–1992. MMWR 1995;44:46–48.
3. Stovall TG, Kellerman AL, Ling FW, Buster JE. Emergency department diagnosis of ectopic pregnancy. Ann Emer Med 1990;19:49–54.
4. Bateman BB, Nunley WC, Kolp LA, Kitchen JD, Felder R. Vaginal sonography findings and hCG dynamics of early intrauterine and tubal pregnancies. Obstet Gynecol 1990;75:421–427.
5. Cacciatore B, Stenman UH, Ylostalo P. Early screening for ectopic pregnancy in high-risk symptom-free women. Lancet 1994;343:517–518.
6. Emerson SE, Cartier MS, Altieri LA, Felker RE, Smith WC, Stovall TG, Gray LA. Diagnostic efficacy of endovaginal color Doppler flow imaging in an ectopic pregnancy screening program. Radiology 1992;183:413–420.
7. Fossum GT, Davajan V, Kletzky OA. Early detection of pregnancy with transvaginal ultrasound. Fertil Steril 1988;49:788–791.
8. Ylostalo P, Cacciatore B, Sjoberg J, Kaariainen M, Tenhunen A, Ulf-Hakan S. Expectant management of ectopic pregnancy. Obstet Gynecol 1992;80:345–348.
9. Shepherd RW, Patton PE, Novy MJ, Burry KA. Serial hCG measurements in the early detection of ectopic pregnancy. Obstet Gynecol 1990;75:417–420.

10. Stovall TG, Ling FW. Ectopic pregnancy: diagnostic and therapeutic algorithms minimizing surgical intervention. J Reprod Med 1993;38:807–812.
11. Karman H, Potts M. Very early abortion using syringe as a vacuum source. Lancet 1972;1:1051.
12. Brenner WE, Edelman DA, Kessel E. Menstrual regulation in the U.S.: a preliminary report. Fertil Steril 1975;26:289–295.
13. Vermesh M, Graczykowski JW, Sauer MV. Reevaluation of the role of culdocentesis in the management of ectopic pregnancy. Am J Obstet Gynecol 1990;162:411.
14. Romero R, Copel JA, Kadar N, et al. Value of culdocentesis in the diagnosis of ectopic pregnancy. Obstet Gynecol 1985;65:519.
15. Maruri F, Azziz RA. Laparoscopic surgery for ectopic pregnancies: technology assessment and public health implications. Fertil Steril 1993;59:487–498.
16. Gray DT, Thorburn J, Lundorff P, Strandell A, Lindblom B. A cost-effectiveness study of a randomized trial of laparoscopy versus laparotomy for ectopic pregnancy. Lancet 1995;345:1139–1143.
17. Murphy AA, Nager CW, Wujek JJ, Kettel LM, Torp VA, Chin HG. Operative laparoscopy versus laparotomy for the management of ectopic pregnancy: a prospective trial. Fertil Steril 1992;57:1180–1185.
18. Baumann R, Magos AL, Turnbull A. Prospective comparison of videopelviscopy with laparotomy for ectopic pregnancy. Br J Obstet Gynecol 1991;98:765–771.
19. Vermesh M, Silva PD, Rosen GF, Stein AL, Fossum GT, Sauer MV. Management of unruptured ectopic gestation by linear salpingostomy: a prospective, randomized clinical trial of laparoscopy versus laparotomy. Obstet Gynecol 1989;73:400–404.
20. Erny R, Campion-Budar MP. Economic advantages of celioscopic treatment of extra-uterine pregnancy. J Gynecol Obstet Biol Reprod 1989;18:930–932.
21. Levine RL. Economic impact of pelviscopic surgery. J Reprod Med 1985;30:655–659.
22. Seifer DB, Gutmann JN, Grant WD, Kamps CA, DeCherney AH. Comparison of persistent ectopic pregnancy after laparoscopic salpingostomy versus salpingostomy at laparotomy for ectopic pregnancy. Obstet Gynecol 1991;77:129–133.
23. Young PL, Saftlas AF, Atrash HK, Lawson HW, Petrey FF. National trends in the management of tubal pregnancy, 1970–1987. Obstet Gynecol 1991;78:749–752.
24. Shapiro HI, Adler DH. Excision of an ectopic pregnancy through the laparoscope. Am J Obstet Gynecol 1973;117:290–293.

25. Berger GS. Outpatient pelvic laparotomy. J Reprod Med 1994;39:569–574.

26. Fayez JA, Dempsey RA. Short hospital stay for gynecologic reconstructive surgery via laparotomy. Obstet Gynecol 1993;81:598–600.

27. Silva PD, Schaper AM, Meisch JK, Schauberger CW. Outpatient microsurgical reversal of tubal sterilization by a combined approach of laparoscopy and minilaparotomy. Fertil Steril 1991;55:696–699.

28. Loffer FD. Outpatient management of ectopic pregnancies. Am J Obstet Gynecol 1987;156:1467–1472.

29. Tanaka T, Hayashi H, Kutsuzawa T, Fujimoto S, Ichinoe K. Treatment of interstitial ectopic pregnancy with methotrexate: report of a successful case. Fertil Steril 1982;37:851–852.

30. Stovall TG, Ling FW. Single dose methotrexate: an expanded clinical trial. Am J Obstet Gynecol 1993;168:1759–1765.

31. Alexander JM, Rouse DJ, Varner E, Austin JM. Treatment of small unruptured ectopic pregnancy: a cost analysis of methotrexate versus laparoscopy. Obstet Gynecol 1996;88:123–127.

32. Stovall TG, Bradham DD, Ling FW, Naughton M. Cost of treatment of ectopic pregnancy: single dose methotrexate versus surgical treatment. J Women Health 1994;3:445–450.

33. Creinin MD, Washington AE. Cost of ectopic pregnancy management: surgery versus methotrexate. Fertil Steril 1993;60:963–969.

34. Trio D, Strobelt N, Picciolo C, Lapinski RH, Ghidini A. Prognostic factors for successful expectant management of ectopic pregnancy. Fertil Steril 1995;63:469–472.

35. Maymon R, Shulman A, Maymon B, Levy F, Lotan M, Bahary C. Ectopic pregnancy. The new gynecological epidemic disease: review of the modern work-up and nonsurgical treatment option. Int J Fertil 1992;37:146–164.

36. Kooi S, Kock HC. A review of the literature on nonsurgical treatment in ectopic pregnancies. Obstet Gynecol Surv 1992;47:739–749.

37. Garcia AJ, Aubert JM, Sama J, Josimovich JB. Expectant management of presumed ectopic pregnancies. Fertil Steril 1987;48:395–400.

38. U.S. Department of Labor: Bureau of Labor Statistics, personal communication, 1996.

39. Brumstead J, Kessler C, Gibson C, Nakajima S, Riccick DH, Gibson M. A comparison of laparoscopy and laparotomy for the treatment of ectopic pregnancy. Obstet Gynecol 1988;71:889–892.

40. Centers for Disease Control. Ectopic pregnancy—United States: 1988–1989. MMWR 1992;41:591–594.

41. Mueller BA, Daling JR, Weiss NS, Moore DE, Spandoni LR, Soderstrom RM. Tubal pregnancy and the risk of subsequent infertility. Obstet Gynecol 1987;69:722–726.
42. Wilcox L, Mosher W. The use of infertility services in the United States. In: Proceedings and abstracts of the 48th annual meeting of the American Fertility Society 1993;S138 (abstract).
43. Neumann PJ, Gharib SD, Weinstein MC. The cost of a successful delivery with IVF. NEJM 1994;331:239–243.
44. Chow WH, Daling JR, Cates W, Greenberg RS. Epidemiology of ectopic pregnancy. Epidem Rev 1987;9:70–94.
45. Shoen JA, Nowak RJ. Repeat ectopic pregnancy: a 16 year clinical survey. Obstet Gynecol 1975;45:542.
46. Hallatt JG. Tubal conservation in ectopic pregnancy: a study of 200 cases. Am J Obstet Gynecol 1986;54:1216.
47. Thorburn J, Philipson M, Lindblom B. Fertility after ectopic pregnancy in relation to background factors and surgical treatment. Fertil Steril 1988;49:595–601.

Index